More Advance Praise for
Stroke

"In this introductory book that covers a broad array of cerebrovascular disorders edited by Dr. Louis Caplan, the readers will glean much practical information. Each chapter begins with a brief case vignette to introduce the topic to be covered, providing a "real world" context that provokes the readers attention. The case vignettes are followed by useful introductory information about the particular disorder under discussion that is not intended to be comprehensive. A short focused reading list is provided so that those reader's whose interest is piqued by the well written chapters can explore more comprehensive information sources. The 26 chapters were written by authors with a range of clinical experience but the overriding expertise and vast clinical experience provided by Dr. Caplan is evident in all of them. The topics covered by these chapters range from the common to the relatively esoteric, but encompass the great majority of clinical problems seen by busy clinicians. This introductory case-based book should provide an excellent first exposure to the field of cerebrovascular disease for medical students, residents and early stage practitioners that will hopefully inspire them to delve more deeply into this rapidly expanding and increasingly exciting area of clinical medicine."

—*Marc Fisher, MD, Professor of Neurology, University of Massachusetts Medical School, Boston, MA*

"No patient is average. Lou Caplan makes the point eloquently with 26 well described and discussed cases. He arrives at the key points and ^ ^ nces with the perspective and wisdom of ^ ^ and science of stroke. I highly recommer.

—*Vladimir Hachinski, MD, . ty F. .0, Universi .... London, Ontario, Canada*

What Do I Do Now?

SERIES CO-EDITORS-IN-CHIEF

Lawrence C. Newman, MD
Director of the Headache Institute
Department of Neurology
St. Luke's-Roosevelt Hospital Center
New York, NY

Morris Levin, MD
Co-director of the Dartmouth Headache Center
Director of the Dartmouth Neurology Residency Training Program
Section of Neurology
Dartmouth Hitchcock Medical Center
Lebanon, NH

PREVIOUS VOLUMES IN THE SERIES

Headache and Facial Pain
Peripheral Nerve and Muscle Disease
Pediatric Neurology

Stroke

Louis R. Caplan, MD, FACP, FAAN
Department of Neurology
Harvard Medical School; and
Chief, Stroke Division
Beth Israel Deaconess Medical Center
Boston, MA

Stroke Service at Beth Israel Deaconess Medical Center
Boston, MA

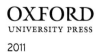

OXFORD
UNIVERSITY PRESS

2011

OXFORD
UNIVERSITY PRESS

Oxford University Press, Inc., publishes works that further Oxford University's objective of excellence
in research, scholarship, and education.

Oxford   New York
Auckland   Cape Town   Dar es Salaam   Hong Kong   Karachi   Kuala Lumpur   Madrid
Melbourne   Mexico City   Nairobi   New Delhi   Shanghai   Taipei   Toronto

With offices in
Argentina   Austria   Brazil   Chile   Czech Republic   France   Greece   Guatemala   Hungary   Italy
Japan   Poland   Portugal   Singapore   South Korea   Switzerland   Thailand   Turkey   Ukraine   Vietnam

Copyright © 2011 by Oxford University Press, Inc.

Published by Oxford University Press, Inc.
198 Madison Avenue, New York, New York 10016
www.oup.com

First issued as an Oxford University Press paperback, 2011

Oxford is a registered trademark of Oxford University Press

Library of Congress Cataloging-in-Publication Data

Stroke / [edited by] Louis R. Caplan.
    p. ; cm. – (What do I do now?)
  Includes bibliographical references and index.
  ISBN 978-0-19-973914-1 (alk. paper)
  1. Cerebrovascular disease–Case studies. I. Caplan, Louis R. II.
Series: What do I do now.
    [DNLM: 1. Stroke–diagnosis–Case Reports. 2. Stroke–therapy–Case Reports.
  WL 355 S918905 2011]
  RC388.5.S843 2011
  616.8'1–dc22
                              2010007931

9 8 7 6 5 4 3 2

Printed in the United States of America on acid-free paper

We dedicate this book to present and future stroke patients. We hope that in some small way this volume improves their care and outcomes.

Preface

Miller Fisher, my mentor, was very fond of saying, "We learn neurology stroke by stroke." Strokes contain all of the elements important for neurologists to learn and know. The neurological symptoms and signs teach localization; the evidence found in hemorrhages and infarcts in a particular region are guides to the clinical picture in patients with other pathologies such as tumors, abscesses, trauma, and demyelinating lesions. The background, symptoms, and course of illness impact on differential diagnosis of cause and pathophysiology of all neurological conditions.

A major unique feature of strokes is their acuteness with the necessity of rapid decision analysis concerning diagnosis and treatment. The last decade has seen major advances in diagnostic technology available to clinicians and development of a larger therapeutic armamentarium. These rapid changes have made it difficult for non–stroke specialists to keep up. This small book with its collection of cases is aimed at bringing non–stroke specialists up-to-date. We included examples of types of problems that are relatively common with a frequency of presentation somewhere between run-of-the-mill daily occurrences and relatively uncommon. We have not included rare disorders. We have emphasized diagnosis and management. When available and germane to the case presented we have included therapeutic trial results. We have also shared our own approach and thinking.

All of the cases have been written by members of the stroke service at the Beth Israel Deaconess Medical Center, Harvard University, Boston, Massachusetts: Adele Al-Hazzani, Ennis Duffis, Richard P. Goddeau, Sandeep Kumar, Gayle Rebovich, D. Eric Searls, and Magdy Selim. I have edited each case to ensure a uniformity of language and format and a simplicity of approach. For more detailed considerations of stroke care consult the "Further Reading" list located at the end of each case.

Louis R. Caplan
Boston, Massachusetts

Contents

Reversible Cerebral Vasoconstriction Syndromes [RCVS], and acute endocrinopathies) and is often referred to as the Posterior Reversible Encephalopathy Syndrome (PRES). The most common clinical findings are: agitation, hyperactivity, loss of vision, visual hallucinations, and seizures.

Stroke

1 Transient Monocular Vision Loss (TMVL)

A 64-year-old man presented to an emergency department because of 20 minutes of a visual disturbance in his right eye that developed that morning as he was sitting and speaking with a friend. He described a "graying of my vision" that started superiorly in the right eye and descended over several seconds to the horizontal meridian. He had difficulty distinguishing his friend's features from the neck up (or any other details in his superior field for that matter). He closed one eye at a time, and confirmed that the right eye was the source of the problem. After twenty minutes, the "gray curtain" lifted over several seconds, starting inferiorly and progressing superiorly. His vision returned to baseline.

His past medical history included hypertension, high cholesterol, diabetes type 2, and peripheral vascular disease. He had never had a similar visual disturbance. Medications included Norvasc 10mg daily, simvastatin 40mg qhs, and metformin 500mg bid. He was not taking an antiplatelet agent.

In the emergency department, his blood pressure was 148/88 and pulse 84. He had a right carotid bruit. His heart was regular rate and rhythm without a murmur. He had poor dorsalis pedis and femoral pulses bilaterally. Ophthalmologic exam showed bright, yellow-orange, round plaques within retinal arteries in both eyes. No hemorrhages were seen. His visual acuity was 20/30 in both eyes. Visual fields were intact to confrontation bilaterally. Otherwise, his neurological exam was intact.

Laboratory testing showed an erythrocyte sedimentation rate (ESR) of 20 and CRP of 0.5. Fasting lipid panel was LDL (low density lipoprotein) 190, total cholesterol 320, and HDL (high density lipoprotein) 30. Transthoracic echocardiogram did not show a cardiac clot or aortic arch atheroma. Telemetry did not reveal an arrhythmia. Magnetic resonance imaging (MRI) brain showed no acute infarct, but a moderate amount of periventricular white matter disease was present. Magnetic resonance angiography (MRA) brain and neck were remarkable for 50% stenosis of the right proximal internal carotid artery.

What do you do now?

This 64-year-old man had transient monocular vision loss (TMVL) due to an embolus from the moderately stenosed right proximal internal carotid artery to an inferior retinal artery of the right eye. Several different terms have been used to describe TMVL in the literature, thereby causing some confusion. "Amaurosis fugax" means a transient loss of vision that can affect one or both eyes. Some authors contend that amaurosis fugax suggests a vascular etiology of vision loss. "Transient monocular blindess" has also been used, but it does not encompass patients who have transient "graying" of vision or partial visual-field loss.

Many vascular and ophthalmologic etiologies can produce transient monocular vision loss. Embolism from the internal carotid artery to the eye's arterial vascular supply is a frequent vascular etiology. This can occur as a result of atheromatous disease or dissection. Cardiac or aortic arch embolism happens less often. Hypoperfusion, retinal artery venous occlusion, and retinal migraine are other potential vascular causes. Temporal arteritis and non-arteritic anterior ischemic optic neuropathy more frequently produce persistent rather than transient vision loss. Eye pathologies such as acute intermittent glaucoma, colobomas, and optic disc drusen may cause TMVL and are useful to exclude by an ophthalmology consultation.

TMVL may portend a benign outcome or may be a harbinger of more serious pathology. Careful history and physical examination, along with appropriate testing, are essential to localize the lesion and determine the etiology. Correct identification of the etiology, and appropriate, timely treatment provide an opportunity to prevent adverse outcomes.

Understanding the vascular supply of the retina can be essential for diagnosing the cause of transient monocular vision loss (Fig 1.1). The internal carotid artery enters the skull base at the carotid canal forming the petrous segment. More distally, the internal carotid artery forms the cavernous and supraclinoid segments. The ophthalmic artery usually branches off from the supraclinoid segment, though it may branch from the cavernous segment. The ophthalmic artery traverses the dura mater and enters the optic canal. Then the central retinal artery branches and penetrates the inferior optic nerve. It divides into two superior and two inferior branches that supply the inner 2/3 of the retina. The ophthalmic artery then traverses the optic nerve. Two or three short posterior ciliary arteries branch off, supplying the superior and inferior optic nerve and choroid. In the case of internal carotid

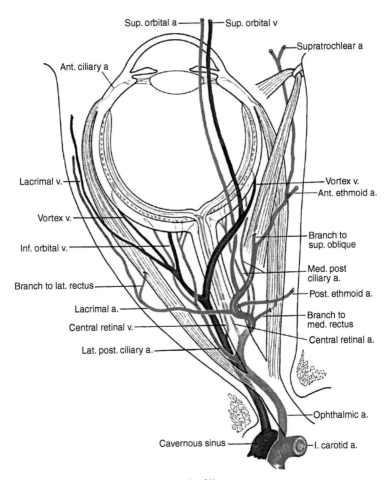

FIGURE 1.1 Drawing of the vascular supply of the eye.
From Caplan LR. (ed) (1995), Brain Ischemia: Basic Concepts and Clinical Relevance, London, Springer-Verlag, with permission.

artery occlusion, the ophthalmic artery may receive collateral flow via several vessels. The external carotid artery may provide flow medially via the anterior and posterior ethmoidal arteries and supratrochlear arteries. Additional collateral flow may come laterally via the lacrimal and meningeal arteries.

Atherosclerosis typically occurs at the proximal internal carotid artery, although it may also affect the intracranial carotid (including the ophthalmic artery branching). Thrombi may form at sites of atherosclerosis. These thrombi may either extend distally, or embolize to the central retinal artery causing TMVL. Dissection of the internal carotid artery may also lead to thrombus formation that subsequently embolizes. If the carotid artery or the ophthalmic artery have severe stenosis or occlusion, episodes of hypotension may lead to decreased retinal perfusion and result in TMVL. Acute diffuse binocular vision loss may be due to hypotension, and is typically associated with pre-syncopal symptoms.

Clinical features of TMVL can give clues regarding its etiology. TMVL is frequently described as a "graying," "blurring," or "blackening" of vision. Often the patient perceives a "curtain" of blackness or grayness that descends or ascends, blocking vision. Usually the visual field that was last affected is the first area to have vision resolution. Partial visual field defects involving only nasal or temporal or superior or inferior fields are possible. Patients may have small central or paracentral field deficits, or the entire visual field may be affected. They should be asked to describe their visual field defects if they close one eye at a time. If a homonymous hemianopsia is present, then the deficit is almost certainly posterior to the optic chiasm. Monocular vision loss is almost always due to a lesion anterior to the optic chiasm. A rare phenomenon is an anterior medial occipital lobe stroke that may cause hemianopia of the contralateral eye's far temporal field.

Altitudinal or lateralized monocular vision loss is most often due to emboli from the carotid because of its proximity to the ophthalmic artery's takeoff. A cardiac source is more prone to cause cerebral deficits. Due to laminar flow, emboli more often affect the temporal retinal arteries, resulting in nasal field defects. If TMVL and contralateral hemiplegia occur, it is highly probable that the ipsilateral carotid artery is highly stenosed or occluded. If a patient with TMVL has infarcts in the contralateral hemisphere or the posterior circulation, then a cardioembolic origin is highly probable. Diffuse TMVL is unlikely to be of embolic etiology, but rather may be due to diffuse retinal or optic nerve ischemia. A pattern of "constricting vision" or "tunnel vision" argues against an embolic event, but could be due to choroidal ischemia. Cloudy vision that persists for hours may be due to retinal vein occlusion.

The time course of vision loss can provide valuable information. A very short duration (e.g., seconds) may be due to papilledema. Patients who have benign intracranial hypertension and papilledema may have brief vision loss if they cough, strain, or change position. Deficits lasting less than a couple minutes are typical of retinal migraine. TMVL due to emboli often lasts one to ten minutes. Persistent deficits are suggestive of temporal arteritis or non-arteritic anterior ischemic optic neuropathy (AION).

Exacerbating factors may indicate the source of TMVL. Retinal claudication describes transient vision loss that is precipitated by bright light hitting the retina and causing ischemia due to poor vascular reserve. Retinal claudication suggests ipsilateral severe carotid stenosis or occlusion. Patients with severe carotid stenosis who change neck position, exercise, or who have just eaten may transiently decrease blood flow to the retina and may have TMVL. Gaze-evoked TMVL suggests an orbital mass or Grave's ophthalmopathy.

The physical exam should focus on the carotids and heart. Is there a carotid bruit? Carotid bruits tend to produce a focal, high pitched, long sound. Is there arrhythmia or a heart murmur that would suggest cardiac embolism? The neurological exam must include fundoscopy. Are there any embolic particles? The appearance of embolic particles within retinal arteries can give clues as to the type and origin of emboli. A blanched retina with decreased vascularity suggests red thrombi from the heart, aorta, or occluded internal carotid artery (ICA). Gray-white elongated particles suggest white thrombi, composed of platelets and fibrin, from the ICA. Hollenhorst plaques are cholesterol crystals that appear bright, orange-yellow, and round (Fig 1.2). They most often originate from the ICA and aorta. Calcium particles are chalky-white and often come from the aortic or mitral valves. Other types of emboli include fat, myxoma, and septic emboli. Is there optic disc swelling? Unilateral papilledema is probably an acute event due to inflammation or ischemia. Optic disc pallor is more likely a subacute or chronic event, occurring at 4–6 weeks. Visual acuity and visual fields must also be assessed.

Patients with TMVL due to a thromboembolic event have a lower risk of subsequent hemispheric stroke than patients who initially present with a hemispheric stroke. Analysis of the NASCET trial found that TMVL due to thromboembolism had a 3-year risk of subsequent hemispheric stroke that was half the rate of patients presenting initially with cerebral ischemia. Risk factors for subsequent stroke include: age greater than 75, male gender, history of hemispheric stroke or transient ischemic attack (TIA), history

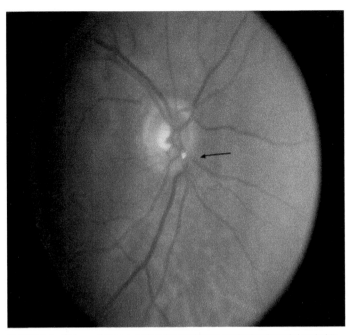

FIGURE 1.2 Picture of the ocular fundus showing a cholesterol crystal embolus (black arrow).

of intermittent claudication, high grade carotid stenosis (80–99%), and poor or absent collateral circulation. In another study, TMVL that occurred more than ten times was associated with ipsilateral ICA occlusion rather than severe stenosis. Retinal claudication also was associated with total ICA occlusion.

Temporal arteritis must be considered because it is treatable and because missing this diagnosis may result in permanent blindness. Temporal arteritis is a granulomatous inflammation of medium and large arteries. On exam, the temporal artery may have firm sections that are not easily compressible. Temporal artery pulsation may be absent. The short posterior ciliary arteries may have arteritic occlusions or stenoses. Vision loss is typically sudden, persistent, painful, and monocular. Transient vision loss is uncommon, occurring in only 10–15% of patients. Many patients have headache, jaw claudication, and polymyalgia rheumatica.

Non-arteritic anterior ischemic optic neuropathy (non-arteritic AION) is a form of small vessel disease caused by optic nerve head ischemia and "crowding of the optic disc." These patients have a crowded optic disc with a small diameter and an absent or small cup. Axon ischemia can lead to axoplasmic flow stasis and swelling. As the axons swell, they compress capillaries in between the axons, causing poor perfusion and secondary vascular changes in the optic nerve head. Higher blood pressure is needed in the capillaries to maintain flow. Nocturnal blood pressure drops may produce additional ischemia and vision loss. One study found that more than 75% of patients initially discover vision loss in the morning after awakening or after a nap. This vision loss is usually persistent and painless. An altitudinal defect may be present. Forty percent of patients may develop AION in the contralateral eye.

Retinal migraine is caused by reversible vasospasm of retinal vessels without systemic vasospasm. Patients have repetitive episodes that are usually short in duration, a few minutes. Reversible negative visual phenomena such as "graying" of vision or scotomata are more frequent than positive phenomena. The patient should have a personal or family history of migraine.

Less common vascular causes of TMVL include vasculitis (e.g., Wegener's or Takayasu's), fibromuscular dysplasia, cocaine-induced vasospasm, and vascular malformations. These vascular malformations include aneurysms of the internal carotid artery at the ophthalmic artery's origin, orbital arteriovenous fistula, and cavernous sinus thrombosis. Hypercoagulable syndromes, especially antiphospholipid antibody syndrome, may result in TMVL. Patients should be asked for any history of miscarriage, deep venous thrombosis, erythema, or family history of hypercoagulability.

The evaluation of TMVL patients should be guided by their clinical features and examination. Patients suspected of having thromboembolic disease, temporal arteritis, retinal vein disease, glaucoma, or other intra-ocular causes of transient vision loss should be referred to an ophthalmologist. Patients older than 50 should be evaluated with ESR and CRP to exclude temporal arteritis. If ESR and/or CRP are elevated, or if the presentation is concerning for temporal arteritis, then steroids should be started and a temporal artery biopsy obtained. Initiation of steroids should not be delayed until the biopsy results are known because treatment delay may lead to permanent vision loss. Color doppler ultrasound of the orbit may be obtained. In patients with ocular ischemia, this may reveal decreased blood velocities, reversal of blood flow, and increased vascular resistance. The advantages are that it is rapid, non-invasive, and gives quantitative information. IV fluorescein angiography is an invasive technique that can be used to visualize orbital arterial flow. TMVL patients who are older than 50 or younger patients with multiple vascular risk factors should undergo MRI brain and vascular imaging. This vascular imaging could include MRA brain and neck, CTA brain and neck, or carotid ultrasound. If no carotid stenosis is found, then a transthoracic echocardiogram may be obtained. Patients who are suspected to be hypercoagulable should have a hypercoagulability panel checked. Treatment will depend on the etiology of the transient monocular visual loss.

KEY POINTS TO REMEMBER

- Transient monocular vision loss may be the result of thromboembolic disease, temporal arteritis, non-arteritic anterior ischemic optic neuropathy, retinal migraine, other vascular causes (dissection, vasculitis, vascular malformations), and ocular causes.
- Transient monocular vision loss occurs most frequently as a result of emboli from the proximal internal carotid artery than from the heart or aorta.
- Patients who have an initial episode of transient monocular vision loss due to a thromboembolic mechanism have half the risk of subsequent hemispheric stroke compared to patients who initially present with hemispheric stroke.
- Thorough physical, ophthalmological, and neurological exams are essential for discovering the etiology of TMVL. Retinal findings may suggest the origin of retinal emboli.
- Temporal arteritis is a preventable cause of permanent visual loss. If there is clinical suspicion for temporal arteritis, treatment with steroids must begin immediately.
- TMVL patients who are older than 50 or younger patients with multiple vascular risk factors should undergo MRI brain and vascular imaging.

Further Reading

Benavente O, Eliasziw M, Streifler JY, et al. (2001). Prognosis after transient monocular blindness associated with carotid-artery stenosis. *N Engl J Med* 345:1084-1090.

Bruno A, Corbett JJ, Biller J, et al. (1990). Transient monocular visual loss patterns and associated vascular abnormalities. *Stroke* 21:34-39.

Caselli RJ, Hunder GG, Whisnant JP. (1988). Neurologic disease in biopsy-proven giant cell (temporal) arteritis. *Neurology* 38:352-359.

Donders RC. (2001). Clinical features of transient monocular blindness and the likelihood of atherosclerotic lesions of the internal carotid artery. *J Neurol Neurosurg Psychiatry* 71:247-249.

Fisher CM. (1989). Transient monocular blindness versus amaurosis fugax. *Neurology* 39:1622-1624.

Hayreh SS, Zimmerman MB. (2007). Incipient nonarteritic anterior ischemic optic neuropathy. *Ophthalmology* 114:1763-1772.

Pessin MS, Duncan GW, Mohr JP, Poskanzer DC. (1977). Clinical and angiographic features of carotid transient ischemic attacks. *N Engl J Med* 296:358-362.

Winterkorn J, Kupersmith M, Wirtschafter JD, Forman S. (1993). Treatment of vasospastic amaurosis fugax with calcium-channel blockers. *N Engl J Med* 329:396-398.

Cerebellar Infarct and Vertebral Artery Neck Occlusion

A 55-year-old Caucasian man suddenly became dizzy while shoveling snow and could not walk. His wife helped him inside. In the ambulance he vomited and felt discomfort in the back of his left head, neck, and shoulder. He had had hypertension for 10 years, and 5 years ago he had coronary artery bypass surgery. He took aspirin, a statin, and an angiotensin converting enzyme inhibitor. Three days before, he had had a very brief attack of dizziness and blurred vision, and had veered to the left. He had not reported this episode to his doctor.

   On examination: blood pressure 155/90; pulse 80 and regular. No cardiac enlargement or murmurs. Neurological abnormalities included: nystagmus on left lateral horizontal gaze; overshoot on rapid ascent and descent of his left arm; tilting to the left when he stood or attempted to walk.

What do you do now?

An embolus had arisen from an occluded left vertebral artery in the neck and had embolized to the left intracranial vertebral artery, blocking its posterior inferior cerebellar artery (PICA) branch and causing a left cerebellar infarct. The blood supply of the cerebellum is strategically located so that parts of the cerebellum lie within each of the intracranial posterior circulation territories. Figures 2.1a and b show the blood supply of the cerebellum. The posterior undersurface of the cerebellum is fed by the PICA branches of the intracranial vertebral arteries (ICVAs), which are within the proximal intracranial territory. A small portion of the undersurfaces of the cerebellum and the flocculus and brachium pontis are supplied by the anterior inferior cerebellar artery (AICA) branches of the proximal basilar artery, which lie within the middle intracranial territory. The superior surface of the cerebellum is supplied by the superior cerebellar arteries (SCAs), which are branches of the very rostral basilar artery, a portion of the distal intracranial territory. MRI scans, especially **T2-weighted** sagittal sections, allow ready localization of infarction to one of the cerebellar artery territories—PICA, AICA, or SCA—and so localize the vascular lesion to proximal, middle, or distal intracranial territory or combinations thereof (Figs 2.2a and b). Analysis of the location of cerebellar infarcts provides clues as to the underlying intracranial vascular lesions and the causative stroke mechanisms. If the infarct is in PICA territory, then the occlusive lesion (in situ or embolic) must have been (at least transiently) at the level of the intracranial vertebral artery. If the AICA territory is involved, then the lesion must have been in the basilar artery or its AICA branch. If in the basilar artery itself, then the infarct invariably involves more than one AICA territory distribution (AICA+). If the infarct is in SCA territory, then the blockage must have been at the level of the top of the basilar artery.

DIAGNOSIS

The cardinal signs of cerebellar infarction are gait instability and ataxia. Vomiting is also common. Since the tentorium and dura adjacent to the cerebellum are supplied by the upper cervical nerves, patients with large infarcts often describe discomfort in the back of the head, neck, and shoulder

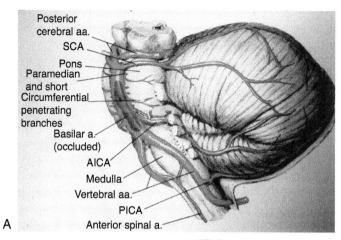

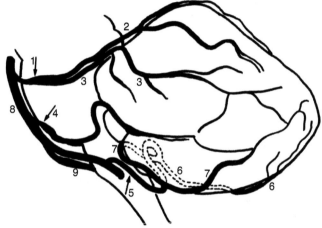

FIGURE 2.1 Artist's Drawings of the Cerebellar Blood supply
a. Artist's (Netter) drawing of the cerebellum and its blood supply. From Netter
FH. (1986). *The Netter Collection of Medical Illustrations. Vol 1 Nervous System*,
Part II, section III, plate 14, p. 64. ICON learning Systems, with permission.
b. Black and white drawing of the cerebellar supply arteries. From Amarenco P,
Hauw JJ, Caplan LR. (1993). Cerebellar infarctions. In: *Handbook of Cerebellar
Diseases* (Lechtenberg R, ed.). New York, Marcel Dekker.
  1. superior cerebellar artery (SCA)
  2 and 3. medial and lateral branches of the superior cerebellar artery
  4. anterior inferior cerebellar artery (AICA)
  5. posterior inferior cerebellar artery (PICA)
  6 and 7. medial and lateral branches of the posterior inferior
  cerebellar artery
  8. basilar artery
  9. intracranial vertebral artery

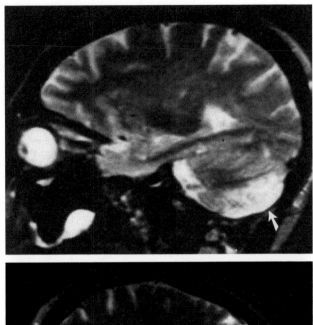

A

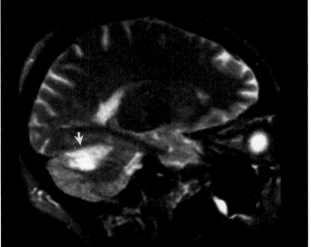

B

FIGURE 2.2 Sagittal T2-weighted MRI scans of the cerebellum. From Caplan LR. (2009), *Caplan's Stroke: A Clinical Approach*, 4th edition, Philadelphia, Elsevier, with permission.

a. Scan shows a PICA territory cerebellar infarct (white arrow) involving the inferior cerebellum.

b. Scan shows show an SCA territory cerebellar infarct (white arrowhead) involving the superior cerebellum.

on the same side as the infarct. When the patient is examined in bed, their motor, reflex, and sensory examinations may appear normal. The limbs are not weak. Finger-to-nose coordination is also often normal when the infarct involves the inferior cerebellum (the commonest location of cerebellar infarction). The most important examination is to watch the patient sit, stand, and walk. Often the patient will lean or tilt to the side of the infarct or backward and may be unable to walk.

Some patients have nystagmus or an asymmetry of conjugate gaze toward the side of the infarct. The other key test is to have the patient stretch their arms in front of them and then rapidly elevate and then drop both arms together halting the ascent and descent abruptly but avoiding hitting the lap. Invariably the arm on the side of the inferior cerebellar infarct will lag behind the contralateral arm and will overshoot the stopping region. The same test is often positive in patients with lateral medullary infarcts that involve the inferior cerebellar peduncle leading to the cerebellum. This patient's findings are typical for cerebellar infarction, and he had no brainstem findings indicative of medullary infarction.

CT scans of patients with recent cerebellar ischemia may be normal or include subtle abnormalities readily overlooked. MRI scans that include diffusion-weighted images (DWI) are more reliable. Often the CT abnormalities appear later.

MANAGEMENT

Treatment of patients with cerebellar infarction concerns two major aspects: 1) monitoring for increase in pressure in the posterior fossa that potentially could cause fatal compression of the brainstem, and 2) treatments related to the causative vascular process.

Large so-called pseudotumoral cerebellar infarcts can distort the IVth ventricle, causing development of hydrocephalus, increasing intracranial contents and pressure. The tegmentum of the medulla and pons can be directly compressed by the swollen cerebellum and the basal portions of the lower brainstem pushed against the clivus. Cerebellar tonsillar herniation through the foramen magnum can compress the lower medulla and rostral spinal cord. Upward herniation of the rostral cerebellum through the tentorial incisura causes distortion of the midbrain and aqueduct of Sylvius with buckling of the quadrigeminal plate.

Important clinical signs of worsening include: a decrease in alertness, bilateral gaze palsies, and Babinski signs. Neuroimaging is essential for the recognition of pseudotumoral infarcts and to identify coexistent brainstem infarction. MRI is clearly superior to CT for this purpose. Obliteration of posterior fossa cisterns is an important sign of pressure development and can be seen on CT scans. Midline shifts, compression or obliteration of the IVth ventricle, and hydrocephalus should be readily detected on both CT and MRI scans. Upward and downward cerebellar herniation can best be shown on midsagittal MRI sections. T2-weighted sagittal sections are especially helpful, since they usually optimally show the localization of the cerebellar infarcts as well as the vertical shifts and herniations.

The optimal treatment of patients with pseudotumoral infarcts is still unsettled. Corticosteroids and osmotic agents as well as hyperventilation are useful in decreasing cerebellar edema in patients with slight mass effect. There is general agreement that ventricular drainage should be used in patients who have hydrocephalus and who have developed decreased level of consciousness and/or new brainstem signs. Surgical removal of dead swollen cerebellar tissue can be life-saving if the more conservative measures are not successful.

Most PICA-territory inferior cerebellar infarcts are caused by embolic occlusion of the intracranial vertebral artery on the side of the infarct. The commonest sources are the heart, aorta, and vertebral artery origin in the neck. Vertebral artery atherosclerosis is especially common in Caucasian men and shares the same risk factors as carotid artery disease in the neck. This patient formed a thrombus that was superimposed on a severely atherosclerotic narrowed vertebral artery. Cervical vertebral artery dissections can also serve as an artery-to-artery source of embolism. Atherosclerotic lesions of the intracranial vertebral artery can also explain cerebellar infarction, but the infarcts are smaller than those caused by embolism.

Management of acute thromboembolism emanating from the vertebral artery in the neck is similar to that of acute carotid artery thrombosis.

When the thrombus first forms it is not well organized and not adherent and can and does embolize intracranially as in this patient. We usually advocate short-term anticoagulation with heparin and later warfarin to prevent recurrent embolization. After 4–6 weeks the thrombus becomes adherent and organized and embolization is rare. At that time antiplatelets can be substituted for the anticoagulant. In this patient a large cerebellar infarct would render acute anticoagulation more risky because of the potential of bleeding into the infarct, potentiating herniation. Antiplatelet agents are an acceptable choice for prophylaxis.

KEY POINTS TO REMEMBER

- The cardinal signs of cerebellar infarction are gait instability and ataxia.
- Large (so-called pseudotumoral) cerebellar infarcts can cause mass effect within the posterior fossa and compress the brainstem, leading to coma and death.
- A change in level of consciousness, bilateral horizontal gaze palsies, and bilateral Babinski signs are early signs of brainstem compression.
- Surgical decompression of pseudotumoral cerebellar infarcts can be life-saving.
- Atherosclerotic occlusive disease frequently involves the first portion of the vertebral artery in the neck.
- Large cerebellar infarcts in the territories of the posterior inferior or superior cerebellar arteries are often caused by intra-arterial embolism arising from vertebral artery occlusive disease in the neck or head, or from the heart or aorta.

Further Reading

Amarenco P, Hauw J-J, Caplan LR. (1994). Cerebellar infarctions. In: *Handbook of Cerebellar Diseases* (Lechtenberg R, ed.), pp. 251-290. New York, Marcel Dekker Inc.

Caplan LR. (2005). Cerebellar infarcts. *Rev Neurol Dis* 2:51-60.

Caplan LR. (2008). *Caplan's Stroke: A Clinical Approach*, 4th edition. Philadelphia, Elsevier, ch. 7, pp. 269-271.

Rieke K, Krieger D, Adams H-P, et al. (1993). Therapeutic strategies in space-occupying cerebellar infarction based on clinical, neuroradiological and neurophysiological data. *Cerebrovasc Dis* 3:45–55.

Savitz SI, Caplan LR. (2005). Current concepts: vertebrobasilar disease. *New England Journal of Medicine* 352:2618–2626.

The Netter Collection of Medical Illustrations. Vol I Nervous System

3 Lateral Medullary Infarction

A 43-year-old Chinese man came to the hospital because he could not swallow. Two days before he had suddenly felt a sharp hot stabbing feeling in his right eye and cheek, quickly followed by dizziness and unsteady gait. His voice became hoarse and he choked when he drank tea. He had been an insulin-dependent diabetic for 10 years. He had had several brief episodes of dizziness during the preceding weeks, once accompanied by a feeling that objects were jiggling (oscillopsia).
Examination showed: blood pressure 135/75, pulse 74 and regular, no cardiac abnormalities and no neck bruits. Neurological findings included: decreased pain and temperature sensation on the face bilaterally and the left trunk and limbs; right ptosis and meiosis; nystagmus on right lateral horizontal gaze; hoarse speech and an occasional crowing-like cough; decreased motion of the right palate; and unsteady gait. Hiccups developed later and were a continued nuisance.

What do you do now?

This man had developed a right lateral medullary syndrome caused by a stenotic lesion in his right intracranial vertebral artery. The stenosis had caused decreased flow in the branch arteries that penetrate through the lateral medullary fossa to supply portions of the lateral medulla. Figure 3.1 is a drawing that shows the occlusive vascular lesion and the resultant infarct in the lateral medulla. The syndrome is so important to recognize that I will describe its components in some detail herein.

Vestibulo-cerebellar symptoms and signs are nearly always present in patients with lateral medullary infarcts.The vestibular nuclei and their connections with oculomotor structures including the vestibulo-ocular reflex (VOR) and the vestibular portions of the cerebellum form a functional unit. Most patients speak of feeling dizzy or off-balance, while others describe frank vertigo. Feelings of tilting or leaning are also frequent. Disturbances in the vestibular system are sometimes manifested as visual symptoms because of abnormalities in the VOR. Patients report blurred vision, diplopia, or oscillopsia, rhythmic motion or oscillation of objects on which they attempt to focus.

Ataxia is a common finding. It can relate to involvement of the vestibular nuclei; the inferior cerebellar peducle, which carries fiber connnections to the cerebellum; or the cerebellum itself. Patients describe tilting, veering, or falling to one side when they sit or try to stand. When walking, the pulling and veering sensations are accentuated. Truncal imbalance is more prominent than limb ataxia. Patients with lateral medullary infarcts initially often have difficulty sitting upright without support. They topple, lean, or veer to the ipsilateral side when they sit or stand. In many patients standing or walking is impossible during the acute period and several helpers may be needed to support the patient in the erect posture. When they become able to walk, patients often feel as if they are being pulled to the side of the lesion. They veer, list, or weave to the side especially on turns.

Nystagmus is nearly always present in patients with lateral medullary infarcts, especially if there are complaints of dizziness or vertigo. The nystagmus usually has both horizontal and rotational components. The rapid phase of the rotatory nystagmus usually moves the upper border of the iris toward the side of the lesion. Most often, the larger amplitude, slower nystagmus is present on gaze to the side of the lesion, while smaller amplitude

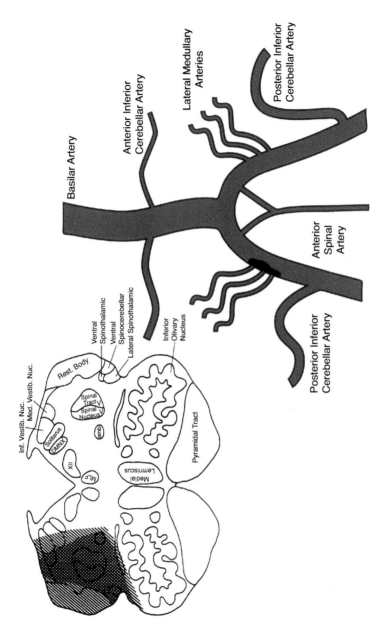

FIGURE 3.1 On the right is an artist's drawing of the occlusive vascular lesion within the intracranial vertebral artery that blocks flow in the arterial branches that supply the lateral medullary tegmentum. The figure in the upper left is the medulla with the infarct shown by dark hatchings.

quick nystagmus is found on gaze directed to the contralateral side. Ocular torsion is also often present with the ipsilateral eye and ear lying in a down position below the contralateral eye and ear.

Sensory symptoms and signs are also prominent. The most frequent location of symptoms is the ipsilateral face. Pain or dysesthetic feelings in the face are often the earliest and most prominent features of the lateral medullary syndrome as in this patient. The facial pain is usually described as sharp jolts or stabs of pain most often in the ipsilateral eye or face. The facial pain is due to involvement of sensory neurons within the nucleus of the spinal tract of V. Numbness or loss of feeling in the face may follow subsiding of the pain. Touch sensation is usually preserved, although patients often report that the tactile stimulus feels different from that on the contralateral face and the ipsilateral trunk.

The most common pattern of sensory abnormality in patients with lateral medullary ischemia is loss of pain and temperature sensation in the ipsilateral face and the contralateral trunk and limbs. This pattern is due to involvement of the spinal tract of V and the crossed lateral spinothalamic tract. Touch, position, and vibration sense are preserved. Usually the loss of thermal sensibility is severe. Initially, the contralateral hypalgesia can extend to the jaw but a sensory level may be present on the thorax or abdomen. Pain and temperature sensibility may be normal in the arm. Sensory levels may appear during recovery. The next most frequent combination is hypalgesia in the ipsilateral face and contralateral face, trunk, and limbs. This pattern of sensory loss is due to additional involvement of the crossed quintothalamic tract, which appends on the medial aspect of the spinothalamic tract and carries pain and temperature sensibility from the contralateral face. In these patients, pain and temperature sensation is reduced on both sides of the face. Detection of the abnormal facial sensation depends on comparing stimuli on each side of the face with the same stimuli on the ipsilateral trunk. Although both sides of the face are hypalgesic, patients note that the two sides of the face feel different and that they are more aware of the ipsilateral facial abnormal sensation. Less often, the hypalgesia can be only contralateral, involving the face, arm, and leg or sometimes only the face and arm. This pattern is due to involvement of the crossed quintothalamic tract and the adjacent spinothalamic tract with sparing of the spinal tract and nucleus of V.

Features of Horner's syndrome in the ipsilateral eye are very common. The descending sympathetic nervous system fibers that course through the lateral reticular substance are affected in most patients with lateral medullary infarcts. Weakness of bulbar muscles innervated by the lower cranial nerves is a very prominent feature in patients whose medullary infarcts extend deeply. Involvement of the nucleus ambiguus causes paralysis of the ipsilateral palate, pharynx, and larynx, resulting in hoarseness and dysphagia. The paralysis of the muscles of the oropharynx results in food being trapped in the piriform recess of the pharynx. Food and secretions have relatively free access into the air passages. Patients try to extricate the food with a cough or throat-clearing maneuver, which makes a characteristic crowing-like sound, probably because of the associated laryngeal weakness. Examination shows paralysis of the ipsilateral vocal cord and a lack of elevation of the ipsilateral palate on phonation. The uvula often deviates to the contralateral side.

In some patients dysphagia and aspiration are the most prominent features. Some patients with lateral medullary infarcts are initially evaluated by non-neurological physicians for primary esophageal disease because of the difficulty swallowing, without recognizing that dysphagia was caused by a stroke. All patients with brainstem infarcts should be carefully tested for abnormal swallowing function. Watch the patient swallow soft solids or water. Formal testing using a modified barium swallow observed by trained therapists is also usually warranted before allowing patients to eat as they wish by mouth. Therapy using swallowing training and modification of the thickness of the dietary constituents can often improve swallowing and help prevent aspiration. Dysphagia usually improves during the first weeks and month after stroke and is seldom a serious long-term problem in patients with isolated unilateral lateral medullary infarcts.

Hiccups are also a relatively common and annoying complaint in patients with lateral medullary infarcts. They usually develop some time after stroke onset but may be present during the first days. Hiccups may relate to ischemia of the dorsal motor nucleus of the vagus or the nucleus of the solitary tract.

Respiratory dysfunction is an important and often neglected aspect of lateral medullary ischemia. Control of inspiration and expiration and their automaticity lies within the ventrolateral medullary tegmentum and the medullary reticular zone. The nucleus of the tractus solitarius also is an important component and is the major afferent input to the control centers. The most common abnormality described in patients with lateral tegmental caudal brainstem lesions is the failure of automatic respirations, a phenomenon especially apparent during sleep. This failure to initiate respiration has been referred to as Ondine's curse because it dooms sufferers to remain awake and vigilant in order to breathe; the alternative is death due to nocturnal apnea.

Autonomic functions are also often affected. Sweating, thermal regulation, and vasomotor control may differ on the two sides of the body. Cardiovascular abnormalities include tachycardia, orthostatic hypotension without cardiac rate acceleration, and intermittent bradycardia. Gastrointestinal autonomic dysfunction includes decreased esophageal motility, gastroesophageal reflux, and gastric retention.

In patients with lateral medullary infarction, the most common vascular lesion is occlusion of the proximal or middle portion of the intracranial vertebral artery (ICVA). Penetrating branches to the lateral medulla arise from the middle and distal 2/3 of the ICVAs and penetrate through the lateral medullary fossa to reach and supply the lateral medullary tegmentum. The medial branches of the posterior inferior cerebellar arteries (PICAs) supply only a small portion of the dorsal medullary tegmentum. The ICVA occlusive lesions decrease flow in these penetrators. Less often, lateral medullary infarction is caused by occlusion of one of the small medullary branches.

When the causative vascular lesion is severe stenosis or occlusion of the intracranial vertebral artery, antiplatelets and statins, and control of vascular risk factors are indicated. Angioplasty and stenting are seldom warranted unless there is severe bilateral intracranial occlusive disease with recurrent episodes of posterior circulation ischemia.

KEY POINTS TO REMEMBER

- The commonest symptoms in patients with lateral medullary infarcts are: pain or dysesthesia in the ipsilateral face, dizziness, visual blurring, and ataxia.

- Symptoms and signs vary depending on the location and size of infarcts. Dysphagia and hoarseness are common when the lesions extend deeply and involve the nucleus ambiguus.
- The distribution of the pain and temperature loss varies, and can be ipsilateral face and contralateral limbs and trunk; ipsilateral face and contralateral face, limbs, and trunk; or only contralateral–face, arm, **trunk**,and leg, or only the face and arm. A **sensory** level on the trunk may be found, and the contralateral arm may be spared.
- Autonomic and respiratory function abnormalities occur and should be sought and treated.
- The most common vascular lesions are stenosis or occlusion of the ipsilateral intracranial vertebral artery, and occlusion of penetrating arteries usually hypertension related (causing smaller regions of lateral medullary infarction).

Further Reading

Caplan LR. (2009). *Caplan's Stroke: A Clinical Approach*, 4th edition. Philadelphia, Saunders-Elsevier, pp. 266-269.

Caplan LR. (1996). *Posterior Circulation Disease: Clinical Findings, Diagnosis, and Management*. Cambridge, MA: Mass, Blackwell Science, pp. 262-323.

Fisher CM, Karnes W, Kubik C. (1961). Lateral medullary infarction: the pattern of vascular occlusion. *J Neuropathol Exp Neurol* 20:323-379.

Kim JS, Lee JH, Suh DC, Lee MC. (1994). Spectrum of lateral medullary syndrome: correlation between clinical findings and magnetic resonance imaging in 33 subjects. *Stroke* 25:1405-1410.

Sacco RL, Freddo L, Bello JA, Odel JG, Onesti ST, Mohr JP. (1993).

Wallenberg's lateral medullary syndrome: clinical-magnetic resonance imaging correlations. *Arch Neurol* 50:609-614.

Intracranial Arterial Stenosis

A 61-year-old Chinese woman came to the hospital
after 3 episodes of clumsiness of the left hand and
slurring of her speech. The first attack was 10 days ago,
when her daughter noticed one morning that her mother
was having difficulties with her left hand and her speech
became difficult to understand for a few minutes. Since
then she has had 2 similar episodes mostly during the
morning, and the symptoms improved within a few
minutes to an hour. She is known to have hypertension
and takes two antihypertensive medications; she has had
no other vascular risk factors. On examination her blood
pressure was 145/80, pulse 78/min and regular, no neck
or cranial bruits. Her neurological examination showed
only slight weakness of the left lower face and deltoid,
triceps, hand, and fingers extensors.

What do you do now?

In this patient, stroke should be the top differential diagnosis because of the patient's age and the presence of vascular risk factors. These recurrent attacks most likely represent transient ischemic attacks (TIAs) that led to cerebral infarction. Atherosclerotic stenosis of intracranial and extracranial arteries remains the most common cause of stroke around the world. The distribution of atherosclerosis is different in white men from women and other races. Studies of African American, Asian, and Hispanic men and all women show a higher frequency of intracranial carotid artery and middle cerebral artery (MCA) stenoses than is found in white men. This variation in distribution of cerebral atherosclerosis in different races is partly explained by the complex interaction of genetic predisposition and racial and ethnic differences in lifestyle and risk factor profiles. Risk factors for intracranial atherosclerosis include diabetes mellitus, hypertension, smoking, and to lesser extent hypercholesterolemia. The ethnicity of this patient and the fact that the preceding transient events were repeated and stereotyped favor the presence of a severe flow-limiting occlusive lesion. The most likely territory involved in this case is the right middle cerebral artery because the weakness is more in the arm and face and because of the possible element of anosognosia—that the deficit was not acknowledged by the patient and was observed by her daughter and confirmed during the examination.

The most common mimics of TIA are focal seizures and complicated migraines. Each could cause repeated episodes. Symptoms of focal seizures and migraine auras characteristically begin with positive symptoms, unlike TIAs, and symptoms tend to "march" or evolve over seconds (in case of seizure) and over minutes (with migraine), while symptoms of TIA are strokelike, that is, maximal at onset. Usually, associated symptoms of migrainous headache or obvious seizure symptoms make the diagnosis easy. The confusion between TIAs and seizures occurs when the seizure is unwitnessed and the patient appears with a focal deficit (e.g., Todd paralysis or aphasia), especially because both could improve over time (minutes). On the other hand, confusion between TIAs and acephalgic migraine can occur, but the latter remains a diagnosis of exclusion. Other differential diagnosis should include reexpression of previous stroke in the context of metabolic abnormalities or infection.

CT scan showed foci of hypodensities in the right centrum semiovale and corona radiate in a stringlike rosary distribution within the internal border-zone region of the right cerebral hemisphere (Fig 4.1). This finding usually indicates an occlusive lesion within the right carotid or MCA. The presence of multiple infarcts within one vascular territory mandate evaluation of the cervico-cranial vasculature to show the presence, nature, and location of occlusion, stenosis, or thrombus within the supplying vessels. CT angiography in this case confirmed the presence of severe stenosis of 90% involving the middle cerebral artery stem. Intracranial atherosclerosis can lead to stroke by one or more of the following mechanisms: perfusion failure, local thrombosis with artery-to-artery thromboembolism, and blockage of flow into penetrating arteries, primarily the lenticulostriate branches of the MCA. Infarcts can be striatocapsular, cortical, cortical and deep, or border-zone, as in this patient. Often different mechanisms coexist and interact. Severe stenosis with limited flow encourages the formation of thrombi that then embolize. Hypoperfusion results in poor washout and

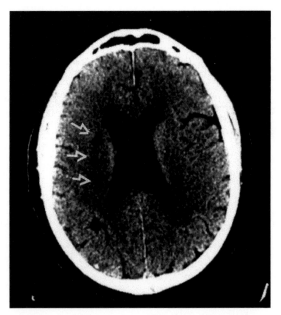

FIGURE 4.1 CT scan showing small hypointensity lesions along the right internal borderzone region.

clearance of these emboli. Necropsy studies show that unstable plaques develop within intracranial arteries just as they do in the neck. When these plaques fissure and rupture, the contents of the plaque reach the lumen and tissue factor is released, promoting the formation of red erythrocyte-thrombin clots (Figs 4.2a and b).

MCA occlusive disease patients often develop their deficits more gradually than comparable patients with internal carotid artery disease. Patients with MCA disease have less frequent TIAs and often note their abnormalities on awakening in the morning or after a nap and usually have subsebsequent fluctuation or progression during the next 1 to 7 days, as in this patient.

Non-invasive tests to identify intracranial atherosclerosis such as transcranial Doppler (TCD) and magnetic resonance angiogram (MRA) are good screening tools. TCD and MRA are useful for excluding clinically significant stenosis, but their limitations are the overestimation of the severity of stenosis and the inability to differentiate severe stenosis from complete occlusion. While CTA shows promise as a screening test for diagnosing intracranial stenosis, still catheter angiography remains the gold standard for confirming intracranial large artery stenosis.

Treatment regimens consists of risk factor management, statins, and antithrombotic therapy. Studies that compared oral anticoagulation to aspirin (ASA) showed that aspirin was as effective and safer than warfarin for secondary prevention in patients with intracranial stenosis. However these studies did not differentiate between moderate narrowing (50–75%) and severe narrowing (90% or higher, as in this patient). Furthermore, patients in whom warfarin anticoagulation was kept within target range had less strokes and infarction than those on aspirin. Patients in whom anticoagulation was below target had more infarcts than aspirin-treated patients, and those patients with INRs above target had more bleeding than those on aspirin. Although antiplatelets should be used in preference to warfarin based on these results, some experts suggest that warfarin may have efficacy in certain subgroups of patients specially those with very severe stenosis, those with basilar artery stenosis, and those who continue to have symptoms while on antiplatelets. Figure 4.2, which shows a red thrombus forming in an intracranial artery, is used as evidence favoring warfarin anticoagulation especially during the acute period of ischemia. Cilostazol is an antiplatelet

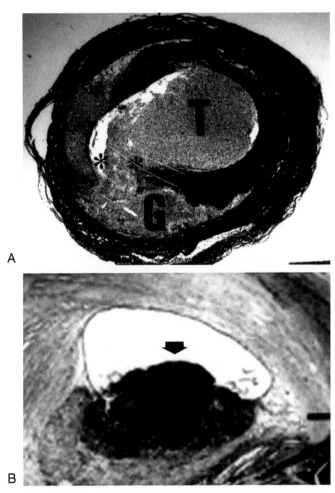

FIGURE 4.2 A Cross-Section of an Intracranial Artery at Necropsy. Courtesy of Dr. Jun Ogata (Osaka, Japan).
a. The contents of a lipid-rich plaque (G) have been brought into contact with the lumen (T), where the atherosclerotic plaque ruptured
b. A red erythrocyte-fibrin thrombus formed in the lumen.

agent with vasodilating and antiatherogenic effects that seems to slow the progression of intracranial large artery occlusive disease when added to aspirin. Dipyridamole, especially in modified release form, also has a vasodilating effect and may be useful in treating moderate intracranial artery stenosis.

Management of hypertension, hyperlipidemia, diabetes, and smoking cessation is a crucial part of the treatment of patients with all vascular diseases. It is important to mention that in an acute setting with symptomatic intracranial flow-limiting stenoses, stroke experts recommend a high normal BP or even hypertensive levels to improve perfusion pressure and prevent further ischemic insult. Target blood pressure goals to prevent the progression of atherosclerosis should be reached gradually over several weeks to months. Finally, endovascular therapy with angioplasty or stenting for intracranial large artery lesions appears promising, but efficacy is uncertain and currently under investigation, therefore it should be performed only in those patients who fail medical therapy.

KEY POINTS TO REMEMBER

- Intracranial large artery atherosclerosis is an important cause of ischemic stroke especially in blacks, Asians, and women.
- Mechanisms of stroke in those patients include hypoperfusion, local thrombosis with intra-arterial thromboembolism; and blocked flow through penetrating artery branches or combination of these.
- The gold standard for establishing the diagnosis of intracranial large artery disease is conventional cerebral angiography but noninvasive methods (CTA, MRA, or TCD) are useful for initial evaluation and screening.
- Antithrombotics therapy and risk factor management are the mainstay of treatment.
- Endovascular therapy with stenting or angioplasty appears promising but efficacy is uncertain.

Further Reading

Caplan LR. (2009). Large artery occlusive diseases of the anterior circulation. In: *Caplan's Stroke: A Clinical Approach*, 4th edition, ch. 7, pp. 221-290. Philadelphia, Saunders/ Elsevier.

Chimowitz MI, Lynn MJ, Howlett-Smith H, et al. (2005). Comparison of warfarin and aspirin for symptomatic intracranial arterial stenosis. *N Engl J Med* 352: 1305-1316.

De Silva DA, Woon FP, Lee MP, et al. (2007). South Asian patients with ischemic stroke: intracranial large arteries are the predominant site of disease. *Stroke* 38:2592-2594.

Gorelick PB, Caplan L, Hier DB, et al. (1984). Racial differences in the distribution of anterior circulation occlusive disease. *Neurology* 34:54-59.

Kasner SE, Lynn MJ, Chimowitz MI, et al. (2006). Warfarin vs aspirin for symptomatic intracranial stenosis: subgroup analyses from WASID. *Neurology* 67:1275-1278.

Mohr JP, Thompson JLP, Lazar RM, et al. (2001). A comparison of warfarin and aspirin for the prevention of recurrent ischemic stroke. *N Engl J Med* 345:1444-1451.

Smith WS, Lev MH, English JD, et al. (2009). Significance of large vessel intracranial occlusion causing acute ischemic stroke and TIA. *Stroke* 40:3834-3840.

Dissection of the Internal Carotid Artery in the Neck

A 23-year-old woman developed diarrhea and vomiting 4 weeks after childbirth. On the second day of illness she had a diffuse headache and felt discomfort in her right jaw and lower part of the face. She noted that her right eyelid was drooped, and she became aware of a whooshing sound in her right ear. It was difficult for her to pronounce some words. Examination showed normal vital signs; the right eyelid drooped, and the right pupil was smaller than the left but reacted to light. Her right palate and right tongue were weak.

What do you do now?

Vomiting had precipitated a dissection of the right internal carotid artery in the neck.

Arterial dissections probably begin with a tear in the media, which provokes bleeding within the arterial wall. Intramural blood then dissects longitudinally, spreading along the vessel proximally and distally. Dissections can tear through the intima, allowing partially coagulated intramural blood to enter the arterial lumen. The arterial wall, expanded by intramural blood, also compresses the lumen. Dissections probably begin from the luminal side at the intimal surface in some patients and dissect into the media. Intimal flaps are often present on the intimal surface. At times, the major dissection plane is between the media and the adventitia, causing an aneurysmal outpouching of the arterial wall. Figure 5.1 is a drawing that shows a typical carotid artery dissection.

Carotid artery dissections usually involve the pharyngeal portion of the artery above the origin but below entry into the skull. Dissections are customarily referred to as traumatic or spontaneous in origin. The great majority of dissections, however, probably involve some mechanical stress. Sudden neck movements and stretching are frequent causes of dissections. Some inciting events are trivial, such as lunging for a tennis shot or turning the neck while driving to see other cars to the side and rear. Many patients forget such events or believe them to be too inconsequential to mention. Congenital and acquired abnormalities of the arterial media and elastic tissue, especially fibromuscular dysplasia, make patients more vulnerable to dissection. Most patients with dissection, however, do not have concurrent disorders. Migraine is more common in patients with dissection. The posited explanation for the relationship between migraine and dissection is that edema of the vessel wall during a migraine attack makes the involved artery more vulnerable to tearing.

Extracranial dissections cause brain ischemic symptoms primarily by the presence of luminal compromise and luminal clot. Dissections through the adventitia lead to rupture into the surrounding neck, muscles, and fascia, a process that causes neck pain and formation of a pseudoaneurysm, but usually does not further compromise blood flow. Thrombus is present within the lumen because of rupture of intramural clot into the lumen or thrombus formation in situ within the lumen. Narrowing of the lumen

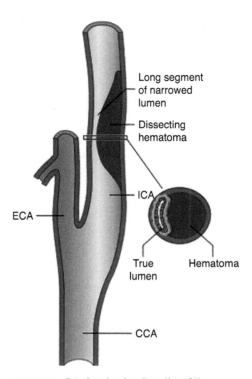

Long segment of narrowed lumen

Dissecting hematoma

ICA

ECA

True lumen

Hematoma

CCA

FIGURE 5.1 Drawing showing dissection of the internal carotid artery The insert is a cross-section view showing the intramural hematoma and the luminal compromise. CCA: common carotid artery, ICA: internal carotid artery, ECA: external carotid artery. From Caplan LR, (2009), *Caplan's Stroke, A Clinical Approach* 4th edition, Philadelphia, Elsevier, with permission.

by the intramural blood, with alteration in blood flow and irritation of the endothelium causing release of endothelins and tissue factors, and activation of platelets and the coagulation cascade, all contribute to formation of intraluminal thrombus. Brain ischemia can result from hypoperfusion (usually from acute luminal compromise), embolism, or both. Hypoperfusion usually causes transient ischemia, but seldom is prolonged enough to cause infarction. Infarction is more often caused by embolization or propagation of luminal thrombus.

The major symptoms of carotid artery dissection in the neck are 1) neck, head, and face pain; 2) Horner's syndrome; 3) pulsatile tinnitus; 4) transient ipsilateral monocular vision loss; 5) transient hemispheral attacks with contralateral limb numbness or weakness; 6) sudden onset strokes; and 7) palsy of lower cranial nerves (IX–XII).

This patient's symptoms are attributable to a dissection through the media-adventitia that causes outpouching of the arterial wall. The distended, dilated carotid artery at the skull base can compress the lower cranial nerves (IX–XII) that exit this region. Figure 5.2 is a carotid artery angiogram showing a pseudoaneurysm of the pharyngeal portion of the internal carotid artery (ICA) that could affect the adjacent lower cranial nerves. The commonest related symptoms are: pain, Horner's syndrome, pulsatile tinnitus, and loss of function of lower cranial nerves. Many patients present with pain and headache as their only symptoms and do not have neurological findings. The pain is often in the neck, face, or jaw. Headaches may be generalized, but are most often on the side of the dissection. Features of Horner's syndrome are caused by involvement of the sympathetic fibers along the dilated carotid artery segments. Pulsatile tinnitus is explained by the course of the internal carotid artery near the tympanic membrane. Patients who present with non-ischemic findings (other then pain and headache) that are present for a week seldom later develop brain ischemia.

Neurological symptoms related to hypoperfusion are usually multiple, brief transient ischemic attacks (TIAs). Sudden-onset strokes are usually caused by embolism of clot from the region of dissection. The diagnosis of carotid artery dissection can be suggested by ultrasound when the ultrasonographer explores the neck with the probe from above the carotid bifurcation to the skull base. MRA, CTA, and standard angiography are helpful. Cross-section fat-saturated MRI scans of the neck in this patient showed a characteristic change in the signal intensity in the wall of the artery.

There have been no controlled trials of medical therapy. In a published retrospective survey, 87% of 572 patients were treated with anticoagulants. Prevention of embolization of thrombus at or shortly after the dissection should prevent stroke and has been the rationale for anticoagulation. Anticoagulants have not seemed to increase the extent of the dissections, a major theoretical concern.

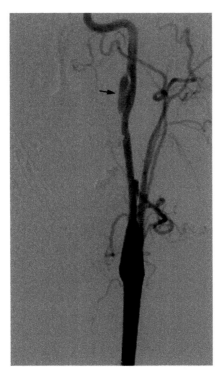

FIGURE 5.2 Carotid artery angiogram showing a pseudoaneurysm (small black arrow) involving the pharyngeal portion of the internal carotid artery.

I use heparin **then** warfarin in those patients who have neurological ischemic symptoms, in those with severe narrowing of the arterial lumen, and in those with intracranial embolic occlusions. The rationale for choosing anticoagulants over antiplatelets includes: 1) evidence that red clot (erythrocyte-fibrin) thromboemboli enter the arterial lumen in dissection patients, and anticoagulants are more effective against red clots than antiplatelets; 2) many reports of others that anticoagulants are effective and relatively safe; and 3) personal experience with more than 200 dissection patients treated with anticoagulants. A randomized trial testing this choice of anticoagulant treatment would be useful, and some stroke experts favor antiplatelet agents. Because the risk of embolization is only during the acute period, I use heparin, followed by warfarin, and try to maximize cerebral blood flow (CBF) during the acute period, to augment collateral circulation. Healing of dissections can be monitored using MRI, MRA, CTA, and ultrasound. I stop anticoagulants after 6 weeks in patients with dissected arteries that remain occluded. I continue anticoagulants in patients with widely narrowed but patent arteries until luminal stenosis improves and blood flow is not importantly obstructed. When arterial blood flow is improved, I switch to drugs that modify platelet function such as aspirin, clopidogrel, or aspirin with modified-release dipyridamole.

Thrombolytics have been given to few reported patients with ICA neck dissections. They might be effective in patients with intracranial red clot embolization who do not have obstruction of the pharyngeal ICA who are seen soon after neurological symptom onset and do not already have large brain infarcts. These circumstances are very unusual. IV tissue plasminogen activator (tPA) is likely to be ineffective when the ICA is occluded. Stenting is rarely indicated, since in patients without occlusions, the arterial lumens usually open well with time and anticoagulants are effective in preventing further thrombi from forming and embolizing. Stenting may be useful in the very rare patient who has severe luminal narrowing and continues to have brain ischemia despite anticoagulants.

KEY POINTS TO REMEMBER

- Vomiting can precipitate arterial dissections.
- Headache and neck and facial pain are very common and often precede other symptoms and signs.
- Neck arterial dissections occur most often in the pharyngeal portion of the artery above the internal carotid artery origin and are provoked by sudden neck movements and stretching.
- Dissections that involve the intima-medial arterial wall often cause brain ischemia, while media-adventitial dissections are accompanied by Horner's syndrome, pulsatile tinnitus, and sometimes signs of lower cranial nerve (IX-XII) dysfunction.
- Strokes develop when thrombi reach the arterial lumen and embolize.

Further Reading

Baumgartner RW, Bogousslavsky J. (2005). Clinical manifestations of carotid dissection. In: *Handbook on Cerebral Artery Dissection* (Baumgartner RW, Bogousslavsky J, Caso V, Paciaroni M, eds.), pp. 70-76. Basel, Karger.

Caplan LR. (2008). Dissections of brain-supplying arteries. *Nat Clin Pract Neurol* 4:34-42.

Engelter ST, Lyrer PA, Kirsch EC, Steck AJ. (2000). Long-term follow-up after extracranial interrnal carotid artery dissection. *Eur Neurol* 44:199-204.

Sturznegger M. (1991). Ultrasound findings in spontaneous carotid artery dissection: the value of Duplex sonography. *Arch Neurol* 48:1057-1063.

Touze E, Gauvrit J-Y, Moulin T, et al. (2003). Risk of stroke and recurrent dissection after a cervical artery dissection. A multicenter study. *Neurology* 61:1347-1351.

6 Intracranial Carotid Artery Dissection

A 46-year-old woman arose and prepared for work. She was found on the floor a few hours later by her husband. She was awake but could not speak or move her right side. Her husband reported that she had complained of a severe headache in and over her left eye the day and night before. There was no history of transient ischemic attacks, migraine headaches, or neck or head trauma. She did not have hypertension, diabetes, or heart disease, and was not taking oral contraceptives. She did smoke cigarettes.

On examination, blood pressure was 130/80 and the pulse was 58 bpm. A bruit was audible over the left eye. She was lethargic and followed no verbal instructions. Her eyes were conjugately deviated to the left but moved fully to the right with oculocephalic maneuvers. She had right lower face weakness, and her right arm and leg moved poorly to painful stimuli. She could not localize painful stimuli on her right arm or leg.

A DWI-MRI scan showed a medium sized left striatocapsular infarct. The MRA showed a severe irregular stringlike narrowing of the supraclinoid portion of the left internal carotid artery (ICA) with extention into the left anterior and middle cerebral arteries. The left middle cerebral artery (MCA) was nearly occluded proximally. She was given anticoagulants and made a good recovery.

What do you do now?

This woman had a dissection of her intracranial internal carotid artery (ICA). Spontaneous dissecting aneurysms of the intracranial carotid system are uncommon in adults, especially when compared with those of the vertebrobasilar system. Intracranial ICA dissection has been associated with fibromuscular dysplasia, cystic medial necrosis, intimal fibroelastic abnormalities, and atherosclerosis. In most patients, no microscopic pathologic changes are noted. The relationship between migraine and intracranial ICA dissection is unclear. One report described a 27-year-old woman who had a long history of migraine, who developed a spontaneous MCA dissection during a migraine attack. Edema of the involved vessels wall during the migraine was posited to provoke the development of the intracranial artery dissection. In another report, 3 of 10 patients with intracranial ICA dissections had long histories of migraine, but all of them reported that the headaches preceding the onset of their ischemic symptoms were more severe than their usual migraines and involved predominantly the retro-orbital, frontal, and/or temporal regions. These locations are frequent sites of referred pain described during stimulation of the distal portion of the ICA and MCA.

Neurological symptoms and signs usually follow almost immediately after the onset of the headaches. This finding differs from that usually seen in patients with ICA dissections in the neck, in which initial pain and headache symptoms often precede the brain ischemic symptoms by several days. Patients with extracranial ICA dissections may have headaches, Horner's syndrome, pulsatile tinnitus, and/or abnormalities of function of the lower cranial nerves without cerebral ischemia (as in case 5). Patients with intracranial ICA dissection almost invariably develop brain ischemia and cerebral infarcts. Fluctuation of neurological signs during the first 2 weeks after symptom onset is common in patients with intracranial ICA dissections and is explained by either intra-arterial embolism or changes in collateral flow due to hemodynamic factors. Cerebral hypoperfusion is the mechanism of many of these events, in contrast to distal embolism, which is considered to be the most important mechanism of cerebral ischemia in patients with extracranial ICA dissections. Past reports of patients with intracranial dissections were mostly necropsy, and they emphasized that most resultant brain infarcts were large and often fatal. More recent reports of patients diagnosed by brain and vascular imaging show that the size of infarcts varies widely and some are small and not disabling. In our patient, the dissection extended to the proximal MCA and diminished blood flow in the lenticulo-striate arteries, causing a striatocapsular infarct.

The typical angiographic findings of intracranial ICA dissection are the same as those observed with neck ICA dissections. String sign, double lumen, irregular scalloped stenosis, and vessel occlusion are found when the dissection involves the subintimal and intramedial layers, and aneurysm formation occurs when the subadventitial layer is affected. The most common intracranial site for aneurysm is the supraclinoid segment of the ICA with occasional extension into the MCA and/or the anterior cerebral artery (ACA).

Subarachnoid hemorrhage and aneurysm formation with mass effect are common complications in patients with intracranial ICA dissections but rare in patients with dissection of the extracranial vessels. The presence of thinner medial and adventitial layers and the lack of a well-developed external elastic lamina in the intracranial arteries have been implicated as the main factors causing subarachnoid hemorrhage in these patients. Most of the cases reported to date have involved the vertebrobasilar arteries, with a few reports describing subarachnoid hemorrhage in patients with dissection of the ACA or MCA. The reason for this discrepancy is unknown.

Some patients with intracranial ICA dissections are misdiagnosed as having vasculitis and are treated with steroids. The diagnosis of vasculitis is often offered by neuroradiologists and is wrong in over 95% of instances of stroke. Among all types of vasculitis with central nervous system involvement, the only one known to affect the distal portions of the ICAs is giant cell (temporal) arteritis. In most temporal arteritis patients that have intracranial involvement, only the petrous and cavernous segments of the ICA are affected, with no involvement of the supraclinoid portion. Giant cell arteritis generally affects a much older population and is associated with an increased erythrocyte sedimentation rate and C reactive protein.

The treatment of patients with intracranial ICA dissection is controversial. Some favor anticoagulation to prevent propagation and embolization of thrombi and cite progression of neurological signs and brain infarction in patients who were not given anticoagulants. Others who argue against using anticoagulants worry about promoting hemorrhagic transformation of infarcts, progression of intramural vascular bleeding, and the development of subarachnoid bleeding during treatment with heparin. In our experience and that of others, patients with intracranial dissections present with either brain ischemia or subarachnoid hemorrhage. Patients who present with ischemic symptoms do not develop subarachnoid bleeding. Patients who present with subarachnoid hemorrhage that have been reported almost invariably have been treated neurosurgically or by instrumentation so that the natural history is unknown. Some probably could develop brain ischemia due to vasoconstriction.

KEY POINTS TO REMEMBER

- Intracranial dissections are much less common than extracranial dissections. Intracranial dissections most often involve the vertebral and basilar arteries and the supraclinoid internal carotid artery. The middle, anterior, and posterior cerebral arteries are less often dissected.
- Headache is a prominent symptom and may precede ischemia and subarachnoid bleeding.
- A higher proportion of intracranial arterial dissections cause brain ischemia and infarction than extracranial dissections.
- Intimal-medial dissections cause brain ischemia and infarction, while medial-adventitial dissections are often associated with subarachnoid hemorrhage.
- Patients present with either ischemia or subarachnoid bleeding. Patients presenting with ischemia rarely develop subarachnoid bleeding.

Further Reading

Chaves C, Estol C, Esnaola MM, Gorson K, O'Donoghue M, De Witt LD, Caplan LR. (2002). Spontaneous intracranial internal carotid artery dissection: report of 10 patients. *Arch Neurol* 59:977–981.

Caplan LR. (2008). Dissections of brain-supplying arteries. *Nat Clin Pract Neurol* 4:34–42.

Chen M, Caplan L. (2005). Intracranial dissections. *Front Neurol Neurosci.* 20:160–173.

Pessin MS, Adelman LS, Barbas NR. (1989). Spontaneous intracranial carotid artery dissection. *Stroke* 20:1100–1113.

Rhodes RH, Phillips S, Booth FA, Magnus KG. (2001, Nov.). Dissecting hematoma of intracranial internal carotid artery in an 8-year-old girl. *Can J Neurol Sci.* 28(4):357–364.

Posterior Cerebral Artery Territory Infarction Caused by Dissection of the Vertebral Artery in the Neck

A 19-year-old college student reported to the infirmary at the university when he discovered that he could not see to his right. During the previous days he had had some discomfort in his right shoulder and in the back of his neck and head. He was an athlete and played on the volley ball and soccer teams of his university but recalled no unusual trauma. He had no past medical ills and did not smoke cigarettes or take drugs of any kind.

On examination, blood pressure was 115/75, pulse was 65 and regular. He had no heart murmurs or rhythm irregularities. A soft bruit was audible over the right mastoid region. Neurological examination was normal except for a right congruous homonymous hemianopia.

CT showed a recent infarct in the left parastriate region of the left occipital lobe. Angiography showed a stringlike narrowing of the right vertebral artery in the distal neck involving the horizontal portion of the vessel after it exited from the vertebral foramina and before it penetrated the dura to enter the skull. The occipital branch of the left posterior cerebral artery (PCA) was occluded.

What do you do now?

D issections usually involve portions of arteries that are mobile. The carotid and vertebral arteries in the neck are relatively fixed at their origins from the common carotid and subclavian arteries. The vertebral arteries are anchored at their origins from the subclavian arteries and during their course through bone within the intervertebral foramina (V_2 portion), and by the dura mater at the point of intracranial penetration. The short movable segments between these anchored regions are vulnerable to tearing and stretching. Dissections can involve the proximal (V_1 portion) of the vertebral arteries usually beginning above the origins from the subclavian arteries, affecting the arteries before they enter the intervertebral foramina at C5 or C6. V_1 dissections are almost always unilateral. The distal neck portion (V_3) of the vertebral artery is the most frequent location for dissection. This segment is relatively mobile and so vulnerable to tearing by sudden motion and stretching as might occur during sports such as volley ball and soccer that often involve sudden neck movements and during chiropractic manipulation. V_3 dissections can extend into the ipsilateral intracranial vertebral arteries and proximally into the V_2 segment. Most often distal extracranial vertebral artery (ECVA) dissections are bilateral even though pain and other symptoms may be unilateral.

Vertebral artery neck dissections were first recognized in patients who had neck trauma or chiropractic manipulation, but dissections have also been reported in patients who manipulate their own necks or who have maintained their necks in a fixed position for some time. Vertebral artery neck dissections also occur after surgery and resuscitation presumably because of sustained neck positions in patients who are anesthetized or unresponsive. These lesions most often involve the V_3 segment.

Pain in the posterior neck or occiput is common, as is generalized headache. Pain often precedes neurological symptoms by hours, days, and, rarely, weeks. Many patients with vertebral artery dissections have only neck pain and do not develop neurological symptoms or signs. Transient ischemic attacks (TIAs), when they do occur, are most often characterized by dizziness, diplopia, veering, staggering, and dysarthria. TIAs are less common in patients with vertebral artery neck dissections compared to internal carotid artery dissections. Infarcts usually cause symptoms and signs that begin suddenly. The commonest locations of ischemic brain damage are the portion of the cerebellum supplied by the posterior inferior cerebellar artery (PICA) and the lateral medulla. Infarcts in these locations are invariably explained by extention of the V_3 dissection intracranially, or propagation or embolization of thrombi into the ipsilateral intracranial vertebral artery. Thrombi within the intracranial vertebral artery block flow into PICA and/or the branches that penetrate to supply the lateral medulla. Sometimes, emboli reach the superior cerebellar arteries (SCAs), the main basilar artery, or the posterior cerebral arteries (PCAs) as in this patient. Young age and presentation with pain and no or minor neurological signs are features predictive of a good prognosis.

Dissections that involve the V_1 and V_2 portions of the vertebral artery can present with cervical root pain. Aneurysmal dilatation of the vertebral artery adjacent to nerve roots causes the radicular pain and can lead to radicular distribution motor, sensory, and reflex abnormalities. Occasionally spinal cord infarction results because of hypoperfusion in the supply zones of arteries from the vertebral artery that supply the cervical spinal cord. Many patients with ECVA dissections have headache, pain, and TIAs without lasting neurological deficits.

Ultrasound examination of the vertebral arteries can suggest the presence of dissection. Typical findings on Duplex ultrasound studies include: increased vertebral artery diameter, decreased pulsatility, intravascular abnormal echoes, and hemodynamic evidence of decreased flow. Color Doppler flow imaging (CDFI) can also show regions of dissection within the neck. Diminished flow in the high neck at the level of the atlas detected by continuous wave (CW) Doppler and decreased flow in the intracranial vertebral artery shown by transcranial Doppler (TCD) suggest the presence of distal ECVA dissections. The vertebral artery locations that have a predilection for dissection are often not well shown on magnetic resonance angiography (MRA). CT angiography shows these segments better than MRA. Dye contrast catheter cerebral angiography is usually able to show characteristic findings. Fat-saturated cross-section MRI studies can show the typical appearance of fresh intramural blood, confirming the diagnosis.

Treatment of internal carotid artery (ICA) neck dissections has been discussed in case 5. The issues are identical to those found in patients with vertebral artery dissections in the neck.

- Vertebral artery neck dissections are common and are often precipitated by sudden neck movements and stretching.
- The first portion of the vertebral artery (above the origin but before penetration into the foramina transversarum) and the distal extracranial portion (after emerging from the neck vertebral foramina but before dural penetration) are favored sites.
- Neck, shoulder, and occipital discomfort are the commonest symptoms and may be the only symptom.
- Strokes are caused by luminal thrombi propagating or embolizing into the intracranial vertebral artery and its branches. The commonest syndromes are lateral medullary infarction, cerebellar infarction (PICA and/or SCA), and hemianopia due to PCA territory infarction.
- Cervical radicular signs and symptoms and spinal cord infarction occasionally occur.

Further Reading

Arnold M, Bousser M-G. (2005). Clinical manifestations of vertebral artery dissection. In: *Handbook on Cerebral Artery Dissection* (Baumgartner RW, Bogousslavsky J, Caso V, Paciaroni M, eds.), pp. 77-86. Basel, Karger.

Arnold M, Bousser M-G, Fahrni G, et al. (2006). Vertebral artery dissection: presenting findings and predictors of outcome. *Stroke* 37:2499-2503.

Caplan LR. (2008). Dissections of brain-supplying arteries. *Nat Clin Pract Neurol* 4:34-42.

Mokri B, Houser OW, Sandok BA, Piepgras DG. (1988). Spontaneous dissections of the vertebral arteries. *Neurology* 38:880-885.

Saeed AB, Shuaib A, Al-Sulaiti G, Emery D. (2000). Vertebral artery dissection: warning symptoms, clinical features, and prognosis in 26 patients. *Can J Neurol Sci* 27:292-296.

8 Pure Motor Lacunar Stroke

A 49-year-old woman suddenly developed left-sided weakness and slurred speech. She veered to the left when walking and had difficulty holding a cup in her left hand. She was an insulin-dependent diabetic, and had hypertension, hyperlipidemia, and an old right cerebellar infarct. Her medications included insulin, simvastatin, baby aspirin, iron, hydrochlothiazide, and lisinopril.

On examination, blood pressure was 157/82; pulse was 89 beats per minute and regular. Neurological examination showed slight dysarthria, flattening of the left nasolabial fold, left-sided hemiparesis, and slowed rapid alternating movements of the left hand. Primary and cortical sensory modalities were intact. She had no visual field defect or visual neglect. She had no bruits. Head CT scan was negative, except for an old small right cerebellar infarct. CTA of the head and neck did not reveal any vascular occlusions. The patient was admitted for further evaluation. Brain MRI with diffusion-weighted imaging showed an acute infarction in close proximity to the right internal capsule. The patient's laboratory studies showed: elevated hemoglobin A1C 10.7%, total cholesterol 228 mg/dl, low density lipoprotein (LDL) 112 mg/dl, and high density lipoprotein (HDL) 97 mg/dl. Transthoracic echocardiogram was normal.

Her hemiparesis worsened during hospitalization.

What do you do now?

The patient's neurological deficits can be summed up as a "pure motor hemiparesis" without associated sensory or cortical deficits. This presentation can be caused by a variety of pathological processes affecting the pyramidal motor pathway, including space occupying lesions, infections, small hemorrhages, or infarctions. The abrupt onset of symptoms in our patient and her vascular risk factors favored a vascular cause for her symptoms, despite negative CT and CTA scans. MRI confirmed the presence of an acute infarction involving the right internal capsule, highlighting the fact that MRI using diffusion-weighted (DWI) scans is more sensitive than CT for detecting early and small infarcts. Pure motor hemiparesis is one of the most common lacunar stroke syndromes, accounting for up to 60% of lacunar infarcts. It is usually caused by a small infarction in the internal capsule or basis pontis due to occlusion or diminished flow through a thickened sclerotic penetrating artery.

Lacunar infarcts have distinct pathophysiological and clinical features that distinguish them from other ischemic strokes. Table 8.1 lists the clinical syndromes associated with lacunar infarctions. Lacunes appear as small, often multiple lesions in the white matter, basal ganglia, pons, and thalami. Miller Fisher, in a series of clinicopathological studies, established that these were due to infarcts in the territory of single penetrating vessels. Fisher and Curry were the first to describe a series of 50 cases of pure motor hemiplegia of vascular origin. They described the presence of a pure motor hemiplegia involving the face, arm, and leg and unaccompanied by sensory signs, visual field defect, dysphagia, or apractagnosia (neglect); and particularly commented on the preservation of mental acuity in the presence of severe hemiplegia as a remarkable feature. They studied 9 of these cases at necropsy, and found that 6 had internal capsular infarctions and 3 had infarctions

TABLE 8.1 **Clinical Syndromes Associated with Lacunar Infarcts**

- Pure motor hemiparesis
- Ataxic hemiparesis
- Dysarthria–clumsy hand syndrome
- Pure sensory stroke
- Sensorimotor stroke (sensory and motor involvement of the face, arm, and leg with complete absence of cortical signs)

in the basis pontis. The location of the infarct causing a pure motor hemiparesis can sometimes be identified based on clinical grounds. Lacunar infarctions involving the posterior limb of the internal capsule are likely to produce a severe hemiplegia equally involving the face, arm, and leg, whereas infarctions in the basis pontis are more likely to be associated with marked facial involvement and dysarthria. Conjugate gaze limitation in pontine infarcts is likely to be toward the hemiplegic side (ipsilateral to the infarct), while it will be contralateral to the infarct in capsular lesions.

Two pathogenic mechanisms for lacunar infarctions have been proposed. These include: 1) lipohyalinotic damage of the small blood vessels due to the effects of poorly treated hypertension; and 2) microatheroma formation within the small vessel wall or at the origin of the penetrating vessel from a larger vessel such as the basilar or middle cerebral arteries due to risk factors such as hypertension, diabetes, smoking, hyperlipidemia, or hyperhomocysteinemia. In recent years, modern MRI imaging techniques showed that a few patients with lacunar-like syndromes have multiple lacunar infarcts on diffusion-weighted MRI suggesting microembolism. In addition, some lacunes are located in the distribution of the internal border zone between penetrating vessels from the cortex and those of the striatocapsular region, suggesting a systemic hemodynamic mechanism. Endothelial dysfunction is likely involved in the pathogenesis of lacunar infarcts, especially in those patients with concomitant silent lacunar infarcts and ischemic white matter lesions.

Recognizing that the pathogenic mechanisms of lacunar infarcts are somewhat different from other ischemic stroke subtypes has important therapeutic implications. Because microembolism is rather uncommon, some have questioned the rationale for using thrombolytic therapy in acute stroke patients with a lacunar syndrome. Necropsy studies of patients with lacunar infarcts seldom shows past thrombosis of penetrating arteries. The pathogenesis of lacunes is thought to be diminished blood flow through compromised thickened penetrating arteries. MRI brain and vascular imaging show that cortical infarcts and large basal ganglionic infarcts caused by occlusive disease of large arteries can sometimes produce predominantly motor abnormalities, suggesting that thrombolysis during the hyperacute phase can be potentially beneficial depending on the nature of the vascular lesion. Anticoagulation is unnecessary and ineffective in patients with lacunar syndromes. In a trial comparing aspirin to warfarin in preventing recurrent stroke, which included approximately 60% of patients who had lacunar infarcts, there were no significant treatment-related differences, and warfarin was associated with a slight increase in bleeding complications, indicating that antiplatelet therapy is usually adequate.

Blood pressure control is one of the most important secondary preventive strategies in patients with lacunar infarcts. In one study, the use of a diuretic in combination with an angiotensin-converting enzyme inhibitor to control blood pressure reduced stroke recurrence by approximately 23%. Similarly, close monitoring and aggressive management of other classical risk factors is advocated. Based on the current recommendations from the American Heart Association and Stroke Council, the target hemoglobin A1C for our patient should be <7%; total cholesterol <200 mg/dl; and LDL<70 mg/dl.

Our patient's treatment was challenging, as her symptoms continued to fluctuate during hospitalization, particularly with positional changes. This phenomenon is common in patients with lacunar infarctions. Blood flow in penetrating artery collaterals is often tenuous and dependent on hemodynamic variables. We kept our patient supine, used intravenous fluids for intravascular volume expansion, and avoided lowering her blood pressure during the acute phase to improve and maintain cerebral perfusion. Her deficits ultimately stabilized.

Although patients with lacunar infarcts tend to have a more favorable functional outcome and prognosis compared to other stroke subtypes, 18% to 33% of patients remain dependent at 1 year. Recent studies have shown that the risk of death approaches 3% and the risk of recurrent stroke 8% at 1 year. The risk of recurrent stroke seems to correlate with the burden of classical risk factors at baseline.

Lacunar infarcts comprise about 20% of all ischemic strokes. The clinical syndrome of pure motor hemiparesis is the most common and easily recognizable of all the lacunar syndromes, especially with the use of modern brain imaging to exclude other pathologies. Recognizing this syndrome in everyday clinical practice is important, as there is a very high likelihood that a pure motor hemiparesis is the phenotypic expression of an underlying lacunar infarction.

- Lacunar infarcts most often involve the basal ganglia, thalamus, internal capsule, corona radiata, and the pons.
- Pure motor hemiparesis, pure sensory stroke, dysarthria, clumsy hand, and ataxic hemiparesis are common syndromes cause by lacunar infarcts, but not all lacunar infarcts cause these prototypic syndromes.
- The commonest causative vascular lesions are lipohyalinosis of penetrating arteries and atheromatous branch disease characterized by plaques or microatheromas obstructing the orifices of penetrating branch areries.
- The most common risk factors for lacunar infarction are hypertension and diabetes.
- Risk factor analysis, clinical findings, brain imaging especially with MRI, and vascular imaging are important in separating lacunar infarction (small vessel penetrating artery disease) from other ischemic stroke subtypes.

Further Reading

Arboix A, Martí-Vilalta JL. (2009). Lacunar stroke. *Expert Rev Neurother* 9(2):179-196.

Caplan LR. (1989). Intracranial branch atheromatous disease: a neglected, understudied and underused concept. *Neurology* 39:1246-1250.

Fisher CM, Curry HB. (1965). Pure motor hemiplegia of vascular origin. *Arch Neurol* 13:30-44.

Knottnerus IL, Ten Cate H, Lodder J, Kessels F, van Oostenbrugge RJ. (2009). Endothelial dysfunction in lacunar stroke: a systematic review. *Cerebrovasc Dis* 27(5):519-526.

Molina C, Sabín JA, Montaner J, Rovira A, Abilleira S, Codina A. (1999). Impaired cerebrovascular reactivity as a risk marker for first-ever lacunar infarction: a case-control study. *Stroke* 30(11):2296-2301.

9 Polar Artery Territory Thalamic Infarct

A 64-year-old academic pediatrician was brought to the clinic in the afternoon by his wife because of a change in behavior. That morning, his secretary noted that his voice was slurred and she saw that he sat at his desk without accomplishing anything. When she inquired, he said that he felt okay. His secretary called his wife, who brought him to the clinic. He had had well-controlled hypertension for about 15 years. He was considerably overweight. In the past he had been hypertensive, and years ago had a basal ganglionic hemorrhage on the right that left him with a slight left hemiparesis.

On examination, he appeared a bit disheveled and had not shaved, blood pressure 140/85, pulse regular. There were no cardiac abnormalities or neck bruits. He recognized and named his physician but could not give the date or the month or the season. He seldom spoke, and his answers to questions were uncharacteristically brief. He could name only 3 childhood emergencies, and 4 zoo animals. He could understand and repeat spoken and written language well but he could not draw the abdominal organs or copy a drawn diagram.

When given 3 items to recall he could recall only one after 10 minutes. His left nasolabial fold was flattened, and his left hand was clumsy. The left deep tendon reflexes were increased, and the left plantar response was extensor. The remainder of the neurological examination was normal.

An MRI scan showed a small infarct in the right anterior medial thalamus and an old right putaminal slit hemorrhage (Fig 9.1).

What do you do now?

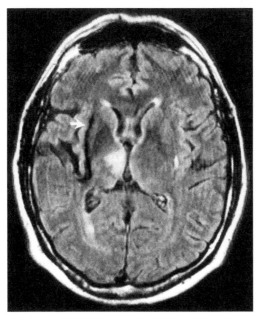

FIGURE 9.1 MRI-GRE image showing an old slit hemorrhage in the right putamen (white arrow) and an infarct in the right medial thalamus in the territory of the right tuberothalamic (polar) artery territory.

This patient's acute behavioral change was explained by an infarct in the portion of the thalamus supplied by the tuberothalamic (polar) artery. The infarct was presumably caused by intrinsic degenerative changes in that artery related to his chronic hypertension.

Strategically placed infarcts and hemorrhages can cause cognitive and behavioral abnormalities that can become disabling, especially for individuals who were functioning at a high level before their strokes. The neurological findings that develop in patients with thalamic infarcts and hemorrhages can be understood by their relation to the distribution of the various branch arteries that supply the thalamus. The tuberothalamic (polar) artery most often arises from the middle third of the posterior communicating artery. In about 1/3 of brains, the polar artery is absent, in which case its territory is supplied by the thalamic-subthalamic artery from the same side. The polar artery supplies the anteromedial and anterolateral thalamus. The dorsomedial nucleus and other thalamic nuclei supplied by the polar artery, including the ventral anterior and ventral lateral nuclei, the medial and anterior pulvinar, and the anterior nuclear group, have strong reciprocal connections with the frontal lobes.

The common findings in patients with polar artery territory infarcts are listed in Table 9.1. Motor abnormalities are minimal or absent. Slight clumsiness or difficulty with rapid alternating movements of the contralateral hand and slight arm drift may be found, as in this pediatrician patient. Facial asymmetry is common, as is a lack of expression in the contralateral side of the face in response to emotional stimuli. Some patients have had minor paresthesias or dysesthesias in the contralateral limbs, as in our patient. The predominant behavioral abnormalities are apathy and abulia characterized by decreased spontaneity, decreased amount and volume of speech, decreased spontaneous activity, and lack of motivation. Lack of spontaneity is often accompanied by lack of emotional responsivity. Some patients do not show emotions and concern for their illness. When directly stimulated by others, they are able to act normally. However activities may stop soon after external stimulation disappeared.

Answers are usually slow and delayed. Spoken and written replies are terse and are not elaborated on. Patients have difficulty making lists of common things such as fruits, animals, clothing, and so forth. Executive functions such as choice of response, inhibition of a response, choice of actions

TABLE 9.1 Anteromedial Thalamic (Polar Artery Territory) Infarcts

1) Apathy, decreased spontaneity, *abulia.*

2) *Lack of emotion* and emotional responses and impaired insight.

3) *Memory abnormalities* especially confrontational recall or recall of lists. Patients with left-sided infarcts have more difficulty with learning verbally presented material. Patients with right-sided lesions often have more difficulty learning visual and visual-spatial materials.

4) Left thalamic infarcts–slight *aphasia* with impaired naming, paraphasic errors, perseveration, with preserved speech comprehension and repetition.

5) Right thalamic infarcts–*left visual and auditory neglect,* sometimes abnormal drawing and constructional apraxia.

6) Slight contralateral facial weakness and slight transient contralateral limb motor abnormality.

among alternatives, selection, sequencing and organizing acts and activities, changing strategies to meet new exigencies, and planning are usually impaired. Memory may be effected, and patients with right polar artery territory infarct may show difficulty in drawing and copying. These abnormalities are similar to those found in patients with caudate nucleus and frontal lobe infarcts. Usually, when thalamic infarcts are unilateral, the abnormalities improve and revert toward normal after 3–6 months. In my experience, and that of others, the cognitive and behavioral abnormalities usually improve with time and are substantially better after 6 months.

The commonest small deep vascular lesions that cause acute cognitive and behavioral abnormalities involve: the polar artery territory of the thalamus, as in this patient; the caudate nucleus; or the genu of the internal capsule. The cause of the infarcts is reduced perfusion due to lipohyalinotic degenerative changes within the penetrating artery branches or microatheromas at the orifices of the branches, or occlusive changes in the parent posterior cerebral artery in a location that blocks flow into the branch.

The findings of abulia, slowness, lack of insight, and altered executive functions are the same as those found in patients with frontal lobe and caudate nucleus lesions. The dorsomedial nucleus and other thalamic nuclei including VA, VL, the medial and anterior pulvinar, and the anterior nuclear group have strong reciprocal connections with the frontal lobes. A series of parallel thalamocortical circuits often also involve the caudate nucleus.

Positron emission tomography (PET) studies have shown abnormal frontal lobe activity in patients with polar artery territory infarcts.

MANAGEMENT

Logical treatment is maximization of blood pressure, blood volume, and blood flow. Because the lesion is caused by hypertension, the most important therapy to prevent new lipohyalinotic disease is to carefully control the blood pressure. Overzealous reduction of blood pressure during the acute ischemia, however, can decrease flow in collateral arteries and expand the region of infarction. I prefer to wait until after the first 2–3 weeks of the stroke to institute major reductions in blood pressure. Blood pressure management is extremely important in prevention of further lacunar strokes. Twenty-four-hour blood pressure monitoring shows that excessively high blood pressures at night with failure to show the normal nocturnal blood pressure dipping is predictive of further development of lacunes and white matter abnormalities. Management of penetrating artery disease also includes maintenance of an adequate fluid intake, and antiplatelet agents. Among agents that decrease platelet functions, the phosphodiesterase inhibitors—dipyridamole and cilostazole—have more endothelial activity and promote vasodilatation and increase cerebral blood flow. Penetrating artery disease and its presentations and management are discussed further in cases 8 and 12.

KEY POINTS TO REMEMBER

- Strategically placed small infarcts and hemorrhages can cause significant cognitive and behavioral abnormalities.
- The commonest such penetrating artery-related lesions involve the medial and posterior thalamus, the caudate nucleus, and the genu of the internal capsule-structures that project to the frontal and other cerebral lobes.
- Infarction in the anteromedial thalamus (polar artery territory) often causes abulia and lack of motivation as the most prominent symptoms. Patients usually improve after 6 months.

- Brain and vascular imaging can identify the mechanism of involvement of the various portions of the thalamus.
- Treatment depends on the mechanism of infarction. In patients with polar artery territory infarcts the commonest mechanism is small artery disease.

Further Reading

Barth A, Bogousslavsky J, Caplan LR. (2001). Thalamic infarcts and hemorrhages. In: *Stroke Syndromes*, 2nd edition, pp 461-468. Cambridge UK, Cambridge University Press.

Bogousslavsky J, Caplan LR. (1993). Vertebrobasilar occlusive disease: review of selected aspects. III. Thalamic infarcts. *Cerebrovasc Dis* 3:193-205.

Bogousslavsky J, Regli F, Uske A. (1988). Thalamic infarcts: clinical syndromes, etiology, prognosis. *Neurology* 38:837-848.

Caplan LR. (1996). *Posterior Circulation Disease: Clinical Findings, Diagnosis, and Management*. Cambridge Mass, Blackwell Science, pp. 413-432.

Lisovoski F, Koskas P, Dubard T, et al. (1993). Left tuberothalamic artery territory infarction: neuropsychological and MRI features. *Eur Neurol* 33:181-184.

10 Basilar Artery Occlusive Disease

Ms. CW is a 68-year-old woman who collapsed while cleaning her attic on a warm summer afternoon. She lay on the floor for almost 5 hours until her husband returned from work. He found her awake but unable to move her left arm or leg; her speech was slurred, though she was able to answer his questions. An ambulance was promptly called. Ms. CW had a history of hypertension, hyperlipidemia, and smoking, which she quit 3 years ago. Four months ago, while vacationing in Mexico, she had a temporary episode of slurred speech and right hand clumsiness accompanied with a headache though she deferred any medical attention. Last week, her right leg was weak on waking up but it improved within 5 minutes, and she attributed it to "a pinched nerve."

Initial evaluation in the emergency room, 5 and 1/2 hours after symptom onset, showed her to be afebrile with a heart rate of 84 beats/minute and a blood pressure of 188/90. She was awake, but markedly dysarthric. The pupils were normal; the eyes were dysconjugate in primary position; she was unable to adduct her right eye, and the abducting left eye had horizontal nystagmus on attempting to look to the left. There was profound left sided hemiparesis including the face; the right arm and leg also were slightly weak. There was prominent limb ataxia on finger-to-nose and heel-to-shin tests on the right, and both toes were upgoing. The sensory exam was normal. Twenty minutes after arrival in the emergency room, her right arm and leg became paralyzed and she was now tetraplegic.

The initial head CT scan did not show any early signs of infarction, but the CT angiogram showed a proximal basilar artery occlusion with preserved flow in the distal basilar and posterior cerebral arteries.

What do you do now?

The patient has numerous risk factors for atherosclerosis and has had two temporary neurological events, very suggestive of transient ischemic attacks (TIAs). The transient attacks involved her right limbs; the present deficit initially seemed to predominantly affect the left limbs, but within a short time all four limbs became plegic. The current clinical presentation showed prominent motor and oculomotor findings with relative preservation of alertness and sensory functions. The current episode started with left sided hemiparesis, facial weakness, and dysarthria, likely due to dysfunction of the corticobulbar tracts and corticospinal tracts on the right; involvement of the corticospinal tracts on the left and cerebellar connections (corticopontocerebellar fibers) produced mild right sided weakness, limb ataxia, and bilateral extensor plantar responses. These deficits progressed due to further involvement of the corticospinal tracts on the left leading to severe bilateral limb weakness. The eye movement abnormality seen here is characteristic of internuclear ophthalmoplegia (INO) implying dysfunction of the right medial longitudinal fasciculus (MLF) located dorsally in the brain stem. The examination, therefore, shows asymmetric but bilateral involvement of motor tracts and an INO suggesting bilateral predominantly ventral pontine involvement with extension to the dorsal regions on the right. These pontine regions are fed by arteries arising from the basilar artery, and the clinical presentation is quite characteristic of a basilar artery occlusion. Kubik and Adams in their classic report on basilar artery occlusion noted that infarction predominates in the pontine base bilaterally and can spread to the paramedian tegmentum on one or both sides (Figures 10.1 and 10.2). This patient likely has adequate collateral flow to the dorsolateral and left dorsomedial regions of the pons, where the sensory tracts and reticular activating systems, respectively, are located, accounting for relative sparing of the sensory function and retention of alertness.

The etiology of the arterial occlusion may be embolic from a more proximal source (vertebral arteries, aorta, or the heart) or from local occlusive disease of the basilar artery. The two prior TIAs provide important clues in this regard. The episode of dysarthria and hand clumsiness and the more recent episode of leg weakness were probably due to pontine ischemia in the basilar artery territory. It is important to note that the patient has not had any vertigo or gait ataxia, which would be more suggestive of vertebral

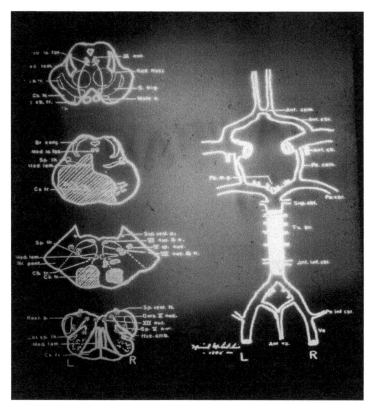

FIGURE 10.1 Cartoon showing the pons with an infarct caused by occlusion of the basilar artery: (a) midbrain, (b) upper pons, (c) lower pons, (d) medulla. Redrawn after Kubik C, Adams R. (1946). Occlusion of the basilar artery: a clinical and pathological study. *Brain* 69:73-121.

artery territory ischemia, and neither did she experience any symptoms suggestive of anterior hemispheric involvement that would argue for a more proximal embolic source such as the heart or the aorta. Dehydration and working in a hot environment probably provoked thrombosis at the site of stenosis in this patient. Previous observational studies have shown that TIAs are common in basilar artery occlusive disease and can occur over days or months. These events serve as early warning signs requiring urgent evaluation and treatment but unfortunately went unheeded in this situation.

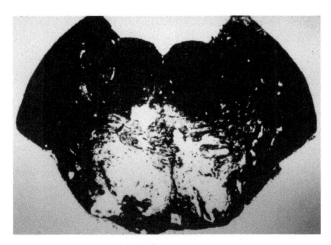

FIGURE 10.2 Myelin-stained section of the pons showing a large infarct limited to the paramedian portion of the base in a patient with basilar artery occlusion. From Caplan LR. (1996). *Posterior Circulation Disease: Clinical Findings, Diagnosis, and Management.* Boston: Blackwell, with permission.

The treating neurologist is confronted with a difficult problem. Almost 6 and 1/2 hours after symptoms started, the patient is severely impaired and will likely have a poor outcome unless an effective intervention is able to arrest and reverse the process. There have been no randomized controlled trials for acute basilar occlusion to aid the physician with decision making. The available therapeutic options include antithrombotic therapy (antiplatelets or systemic anticoagulation), intravenous or intra-arterial thrombolysis, transluminal angioplasty and stenting, mechanical thrombectomy, or a combination of these modalities. The efficacy of some of these therapies was recently investigated in a large prospective multicenter observational study on acute basilar artery occlusion (Basilar Artery International Cooperation Study [BASICS]). Among the 619 patients with acute basilar occlusion entered in this international registry, almost 50% were treated with intra-arterial thrombolysis (IAT), 20% with intravenous thrombolysis (IVT) including subsequent IAT, and 30% with antithrombotic agents. None of the treatment options were found to be superior to the others, although patients with mild to moderate deficits fared better with IVT compared to IAT. The major limitation of this study lay in the potential selection bias for assigning treatments to different patients based on the clinical judgment of the treating physician. For example, patients believed to have a poorer prognosis may have been treated more aggressively with IAT, diminishing the overall efficacy of IAT. Patients in the intra-arterial group also had significant delays in treatment, which may have obscured a potentially beneficial effect of this modality.

The physician who treated this patient opted to initially use intravenous tPA; some improvement in the patient's right sided motor functions were noted. She was then taken for **intra-arterial thrombolysis** (IAT) and observed to have near occlusive thrombosis of the proximal basilar artery with prominent collateral flow through the posterior inferior cerebellar arteries and the superior cerebellar arteries. IAT successfully recanalized the vessel. One month after the event the patient had made a good recovery and had mild residual dysarthria, mild right sided weakness and some arm clumsiness.

KEY POINTS TO REMEMBER

- Basilar artery occlusion is most often heralded by TIAs, which can occur over days, weeks, or months.
- The most common deficit after basilar artery occlusion is a hemiparesis accompanied by slight involvement of the contralateral limbs. Infarcts most often affect the pontine base bilaterally and may spread to the paramedian tegmentum on one or both sides.
- Tegmental signs such as an internuclear opthalmoplegia are most helpful in arriving at a clinical diagnosis.
- CT scans are often not diagnostic soon after pontine infarction.
- Prognosis depends heavily on revascularization of the brain stem, either by iatrogenic opening of the basilar artery (by thrombolysis or clot extraction) or by development of adequate collateral circulation. The brain stem seems to be more resistant to infarction than other brain regions.

Further Reading

Arnold M, Nedeltchev K, Schroth G, Baumgartner R, Remonda L, Loher T, Stepper F, Sturzenegger M, Schuknecht B, and Mattle H. (2004). Clinical and radiological predictors of recanalisation and outcome of 40 patients with acute basilar artery occlusion treated with intra-arterial thrombolysis. *J Neurol Neurosurg Psychiatry* 75: 857–862.

Caplan LR. (1996). Basilar artery occlusive disease. In: *Posterior Circulation Disease: Clinical Findings, Diagnosis and Management, Blackwell Science* 324–380.

Kubik CS, Adams RD. (1946). Occlusion of the basilar artery: a clinical and pathological study. *Brain* 69: 6-121.

Lindsberg PJ, Mattle HP. (2006). Therapy of basilar artery occlusion: a systematic analysis comparing intra-arterial and intravenous thrombolysis. *Stroke* 37: 922–928.

Schonewille WJ, Wijman CA, Michel P, Rueckert CM, Weimar C, Mattle HP, Engelter ST, Tanne D, Muir KW, Molina CA, Thijs V, Audebert H, Pfefferkorn T, Szabo K, Lindsberg PJ, de Freitas G, Kappelle LJ, Algra A; BASICS study group. (2009, Aug.). Treatment and outcomes of acute basilar artery occlusion in the Basilar Artery International Cooperation Study (BASICS): a prospective registry study. *Lancet Neurol* 2009 8(8):724-730.

11 Embolism to the Top-of-the-Basilar Artery

A 52-year-old woman was unarousable one morning.
She had no history of heart disease or strokes.
She reported occasional palpitations and had nearly
fainted during exertion on 2 occasions in the preceding
weeks.

On examination later that day: blood pressure 130/75,
pulse 80 and regular. No heart or neck murmurs or
bruits. She was stuporous and did not open her eyes to
voice or pinch. The right pupil was 2 mm and did not
react to light; the left pupil was 4 mm and had a small
and transient reaction to light. The eyes were skewed
with the left eye placed slightly down. There was no
vertical gaze to doll's eye maneuvers. All limbs moved to
pinch, but the right arm and leg responded less well than
the left. Studies in the hospital showed that she had a
small left atrial myxoma that was surgically removed.

Her husband brought her for consultation months
later because of behavioral abnormalities. She had
uncontrolled spells of crying and laughing. She was
apathetic and had no motivation for any activity but was
content to sit and was uninterested in helping at home or

doing any activity. She slept when not stimulated.
At times she could quickly and even meticulously clean the kitchen and cook a complex meal. When taken shopping she bought and ate junk foods and cookies and her weight had increased.

On examination, she was alert, but her voice was very hypophonic and dysarthric. Her answers to queries were delayed and brief but accurate. Language and naming were normal. Up and down gaze was severely limited. On horizontal gaze to either side the adducted eyes hyperadducted, and abduction was limited. She could not recall any of 3 objects told to her 5 minutes before. She showed a pseudobulbar increase in laughing and crying. She had some clumsiness in the right arm and hand, and pain and temperature sensations were reduced in the right limbs and trunk. She kept her right arm stiff and flexed.

What do you do now?

This patient had had an embolus to the rostral portion of the basilar artery causing infarction in the thalamus and midbrain. Occlusion of the rostral portion of the basilar artery can cause ischemia of the midbrain and thalami as well as the temporal and occipital lobe cerebral hemispheral territories supplied by the posterior cerebral arteries (PCAs). In some patients infarction is limited to either brainstem or hemispheral structures. The major abnormalities associated with rostral brainstem infarction relate to abnormalities of alertness, behavior, memory, and oculomotor and pupillary functions.

The thalamic-subthalamic (thalamoperforating) arteries arise from the proximal portion of the peduncular segment of the posterior cerebral arteries (PCAs). The thalamic-subthalamic arteries supply the posteromedial thalamus in the region of the posterior commissure and the thalamic-midbrain junction. Occlusion of these arteries causes: stupor, amnesia, and vertical gaze palsies. The superior cerebellar arteries (SCAs) located near the basilar artery bifurcation supply the dorsolateral region of the caudal 2/3 of the midbrain by penetrating branches that course around the midbrain. The rostral midbrain is also supplied by direct branches from the basilar bifurcation and the PCAs. The most proximal portion of the PCAs give off paramedian mesencephalic artery branches, and then peduncular penetrating branches originate from the P_2 portion of the PCAs after the entry of the posterior communicating arteries. This patient had infarction of the ventral paramedian thalami, the polar artery territory of the left thalamus, and portions of the left rostral midbrain tegmentum and base as a result of the top-of-the-basilar embolus.

SYMPTOMS AND SIGNS IN TOP-OF-THE BASILAR TERRITORY INFARCTION

In patients with top-of-the-basilar infarcts, the major abnormalities of eye position and movement involve vertical gaze and convergence. Vertical gaze pathways converge on the periaqueductal grey region just below the collicular plate near the posterior commissure and the interstitial nucleus of Cajal. There is a cluster of neurons in this region that is located among the fibers of the medial longitudinal fasciculus (MLF) that are important in vertical gaze. These neurons are usually referred to as the rostral interstitial nucleus of the MLF. Some patients lose all voluntary and reflex vertical eye movements, but in some patients reflex movements are preserved despite loss of voluntary vertical eye movements. Oculomotor afferents that carry information for upgaze emanating from the rostral interstitial nucleus of the MLF and the interstitial nucleus of Cajal decussate from one side of the brain to the other in the posterior commissure, explaining why a lesion in the posterior commissure causes an upgaze palsy affecting both eyes.

Asymmetric or unilateral lesions in the midbrain tegmentum and posterior thalami can cause ocular tilt reactions that are contraversive, that is, the contalateral eye and ear are down. The abnormalities include skew deviation, ocular torsion, and abnormalities of estimation of the visual vertical. Convergence abnormalities are also very common in patients with rostral midbrain lesions. Usually one or both eyes are hyperconverged as if there was increased tone or overactivity of structures that subserve coordination of bilateral ocular adduction called convergence. Increased convergence can be unilateral or bilateral so that one or both eyes may rest inward or down and inward at rest. On attempted upgaze, the eyes may show adductor contractions causing convergence movements. The increased tone and activity of adductor movements is probably responsible for the so-called pseudosixth phenomenon that this patient showed. This term has been used to describe failure of full abduction on lateral gaze in patients with upper brainstem lesions in the absence of a lesion that could affect the sixth nerve. Pseudosixth palsy can be unilateral or bilateral. Close inspection of eye movements in the abducting eye shows that there are often inward-directed small movements of the eye as it abducts. Often the contralateral eye is hyperadducted. Covering the contralateral hyperadducted eye and asking the patient to look further laterally sometimes enables further abduction excursion of the open eye. Two different phenomena explain the failure of ocular abduction in this syndrome: 1) dysconjugate gaze with fixation by the hyperadducted eye. When the patient looks laterally, they first fixate with the hyperadducted eye. This fixation will stop any further lateral eye movement, since the patient has already fixated on the object with the adducted eye. Covering the hyperadducted eye then encourages fixation with the abducting eye. And 2) convergence vectors counter and neutralize the lateral excursion of the eye. The sum of the laterally directed gaze vector and the inwardly directed convergence vector is less than full abduction.

The light reflex arc traverses the upper brainstem with fibers leaving the optic tract to synapse with the Edinger-Westphal nucleus in the midbrain. Lesions in the rostral brainstem often affect the papillary light reflex so that the pupils react slowly and incompletely, or not at all, to light. The pupils are often small at rest in patients with diencephalic lesions and may be fixed and dilated if the lesions involve the third nerve Edinger-Westphal nuclei. A combination of diencephalic and midbrain lesions causes midposition fixed pupils.

Lesions of the reticular activating system in the rostral brainstem produce hypersomnolence rather than coma. The reticular activating system courses through the tegmental regions on either side of the sylvian aqueduct and the banks of the third ventricle. In this region they are perfused by the thalamic-subthalamic arteries and the paramedian mesencephalic arteries.

When patients with rostral brainstem infarcts that include the thalamus awaken from stupor, they may have prominent and sometimes persistent deficits in memory function. The amnestic deficits involve both anterograde and retrograde memory dysfunction, usually including both verbal and nonverbal memory items. Patients with left thalamic infarcts have more difficulty with memory for language-related activities, while patients with right thalamic lesions have had more difficulty with visual-spatial memory tasks. Patients with polar territory infarcts show decreased spontaneity and abulia. They have difficulty generating lists of common objects, for example, colors, items of clothing, fruits, vegetables, cities in their state, and so forth. As in other anatomical regions, abulia and amnesia are usually less severe and less persistent when the lesions are unilateral than when bilateral.

ETIOLOGY

Most often emboli arise from the heart, aorta, or proximal vertebrobasilar arterial system. Particles that can traverse the intracranial vertebral arteries usually reach the distal basilar artery, since the basilar artery has a wider diameter at its origin than at its rostral bifurcation. The penetrating branches of the rostral basilar artery are prime recipients of the emboli.

In this case, the source of the embolus was a cardiac myxoma. Although cardiac tumors are rare, they are an important cause of embolism and are very important to diagnose. The cells of origin for myxomas are endocardial and arise from multipotential mesenchymal cells that persist as embryonal remnants during septation of the heart. About 75% form in the left atrium and 15–20% in the right atrium; and the rest are located in the ventricles and very rarely (<2%) on a heart valve. Most myxomas originate from the interatrial septum at the edge of the fossa ovalis, but some originate from the posterior or anterior atrial walls or the auricular appendage. Myxomas project from their endocardial attachments into cardiac chambers. Embolism occurs in 30–50% of patients who harbor cardiac myxomas and may be the presenting manifestation. Most emboli arise from the left atrium and go to the brain or systemic organs. The most common recognized recipient site of embolism is the brain. Most often, patients with brain embolism present with a sudden onset focal neurologic deficit. Transient neurological deficits sometimes occur. Often there has been more than one brain embolism before atrial myxomas are diagnosed. Patients may also present with systemic symptoms (e.g., low grade fever, myalgia, night sweats) or with syncope/presyncope if the myxoma is large enough to obstruct mitral valve inflow. The woman in this case had transient spells of faintness likely related to temporary blockage of the mitral valve. Usually the diagnosis of myxomas is made when the patient is referred for an echocardiogram to evaluate a suspected cardiac source of embolism. Transesophageal echocardiography is very sensitive for the detection of myxomas.

Occasional patients with brain emboli from myxomas have subarachnoid or intracerebral hemorrhage. Bleeding is related to the development of hemorrhagic infarction or rupture of aneurysms. Embolism of myxoma tissue to the wall of brain arteries causes aneurysms that are similar to mycotic aneurysms found in patients with bacterial endocarditis. Usually the aneurysms are relatively small, multiple, and on peripheral branches of brain arteries. Some aneurysms are quite large. The peripheral location of aneurysms in patients with myxomas and endocarditis differs from that usually found in patients with saccular (berry) aneurysms.

- Emboli that reach the posterior circulation arteries from the heart or aorta that are small enough to pass through the intracranial vertebral arteries, most often reach the basilar artery bifurcation (the top-of-the-basilar).

- Top-of-the-basilar artery emboli can cause infarction in the superior cerebellum, occipital-temporal lobes in the territory of the posterior cerebral arteries, or in the paramedian midbrain and thalami in the territory of penetrating arteries that arise from the basilar artery bifurcation and proximal portion of the posterior cerebral arteries.

- Pupillary abnormalities, vertical gaze palsies, dysmemory, and increased somnolence are typical features of the top-of-the-basilar syndrome.

- Cardiac myxomas can cause episodes of syncope, unexplained fever, and systemic embolism in addition to brain embolism.

- Myxomatous material can embolize to brain arteries, causing distal aneurysms identical to those found in patients with bacterial endocarditis.

Further Reading

Caplan L. (1980). Top of the basilar syndrome: Selected clinical aspects. *Neurology* 30:72-79.

Caplan LR. (1996). Posterior Circulation Disease: Clinical Findings, Diagnosis, and Management. Boston: Blackwell Scientific.

Caplan LR., Manning WJ. (eds.). (2006). *Brain Embolism*. New York: Informa Healthcare.

Mehler MF. (1988). The neuro-ophthalmologic spectrum of the rostral basilar artery syndrome. *Arch Neurol* 45:966-971.

Voetsch B, DeWitt LD, Pessin MS, Caplan LR. (2004). Basilar artery occlusive disease in the New England Medical Center Posterior Circulation Registry. *Arch Neurol* 61:496-504.

Binswanger Disease

A 73-year-old man is referred to a neurologist because of falls and decreased ability to care for himself. He is a widower and lived alone for 2 years. He has had hypertension since age 50. Eight years ago he had a "small" stroke: characterized by sudden onset of left limb weakness that improved considerably during the succeeding weeks. Three years ago his right limbs were temporarily weak. Now, his daughter is concerned because recently he seems more apathetic. He is unconcerned about his appearance. His house is in disarray and looks uncared for. His walking is unsteady, and he has had a number of falls. She feels he can no longer care for himself.

On examination, blood pressure 165/90, pulse 84 and regular. No cardiac murmurs or neck bruits. His voice is low in volume and slightly slurred. **He is alert**. Language and memory are preserved. He seldom initiates conversation and his replies to queries are brief. He cannot give a coherent account of his daily activities or describe any book that he has recently read. His jaw and facial reflexes are increased. He has some difficulty swallowing water and briefly chokes. His limbs are strong but show increased tone to passive movement. The deep tendon reflexes are increased bilaterally but more on the left. The plantar responses are bilaterally extensor. His gait is stiff, and his steps are small. Sensory examination is normal.

An MRI scan shows several lacunes and extensive white matter abnormalities. The ventricles are enlarged, and there is a loss of cerebral white matter.

What do you do now?

This patient has vascular dementia due to chronic microvascular disease. This entity, described originally by Otto Binswanger, a German pathologist, is characterized pathologically by multiple lacunar infarcts and confluent areas of soft, puckered, and granular tissue in the cerebral and cerebellar white matter. The white matter lesions are patchy and predominantly affect the periventricular white matter, especially anteriorly and close to the surface of the ventricles. The volume of white matter is reduced, but the cortex is generally spared. The ventricles are enlarged as a result of the white matter loss. The white matter abnormalities surrounding the ventricles reduce the strength of the supporting tissue and allow more ventricular distention. Figure 12.1 is a necropsy specimen of a Binswanger patient showing multiple lacunar infarcts and white matter softening. Microscopic study shows myelin pallor. Usually, the myelin pallor is not homogeneous, but islands of decreased myelination are surrounded by normal tissue. Figure 12.2 shows a stained specimen showing large regions of white matter pallor. Gliosis is prominent in zones of myelin pallor.

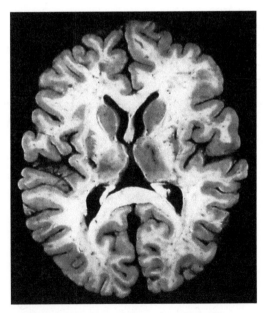

FIGURE 12.1 Necropsy specimen of a patient with Binswanger's showing multiple lacunar deep infarcts and regions of white matter softening.

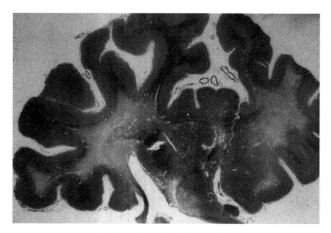

FIGURE 12.2 Hematoxylin and Eosin stained section showing large areas of myelin pallor.

MRI scans show prominent white matter abnormalities and thinning of the white matter (Fig 12.3).

The walls of penetrating arteries are thickened and hyalinized, but occlusion of small arteries is rare. The commonest cause is chronic hypertension, but occasional patients with Binswanger white matter changes have had amyloid angiopathy as the underlying vascular pathology. In these patients, arteries within the cerebral cortex and leptomeninges are thickened and contain a congophilic amyloid-staining substance. Arteries within the white matter and basal ganglia are also concentrically thickened but contain no amyloid. In occasional patients, a granulomatous arteritis complicates amyloid angiopathy. Similar microangiopathic abnormalities in the cerebral white matter and lacunar infarcts are found in CADASIL (cerebral autosomal dominant arteriopathy with subcortical infarcts). The white matter abnormalities appear early. Relatives of patients with clinical CADASIL can show white matter abnormalities before symptoms develop. Usually localized, often nodular focal white matter lesions are found early in the course of illness. Later the white matter abnormalities become more diffuse, especially in the occipital and frontal periventricular white matter. White matter lesions in the external capsule and anterior temporal lobes are particularly characteristic of CADASIL. Occasionally a high hematocrit is the underlying cause or is an important factor. Cerebral amyloid angiopathy

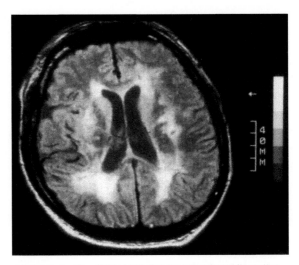

FIGURE 12.3 T2-weighted MRI showing extensive white matter abnormalities and loss of white matter volume.

can cause similar white matter abnormalities but is usually accompanied by areas of bleeding.

CLINICAL FINDINGS

Most patients have abnormalities of cognitive function and behavior. They often become slow and abulic. Executive functions such as planning and performing sequential tasks are predominantly affected. Memory loss, aphasic abnormalities, and visuospatial dysfunction are found less often. Pseudobulbar dysarthria and dyspagia, pyramidal signs, and gait abnormalities are common. The clinical findings often progress gradually or stepwise, with worsening during periods of days to weeks. There may be long plateau periods of stability of the findings. Most patients also have had acute lacunar strokes.

PATHOGENESIS OF THE LESIONS

The mechanism of lacunar infarcts in the territory of a single penetrating artery is clear. The compromised penetrating artery has a reduced luminal size; further luminal compromise by plaque, microdissection, or thrombus diminishes blood flow in the brain region supplied by that penetrator. Hemorrheological abnormalities can reduce flow in that penetrator enough to cause an infarct. Fibrinogen levels are abnormally high in Binswanger patients, and this and low fluid volumes could increase whole blood viscosity and decrease flow through already compromised penetrating arteries.

The two most often posited mechanisms of white matter abnormalities larger than the territory of a single penetrator involve ischemia or increased vascular permeability. 1) Ischemia related to tandem penetrating arterial lesions. This explanation posits severe flow limiting luminal compromise involving a number of parallel penetrating arteries. Hemorrheological changes or periods of reduced blood flow that further reduce cerebral perfusion could produce ischemia and white matter damage in an area supplied by the group of compromised arteries. Cerebral blood flow reduction could be caused by: decreased blood pressure, low cardiac output, low blood volume, or increased whole blood viscosity. Alternatively, blockage of a single penetrator that had previously supplied blood to a region of previously blocked penetrators could produce a sizable area of ischemia. 2) Increased vascular permeability. Leakage of fluid, transudation, could occur when blood pressure within penetrating arteries is very high. Leakage could also occur because of abnormal vascular permeability related to damage or infiltration of the walls of the penetrating arteries. Matrix metalloproteinases disrupt the blood-brain barrier by degrading tight junction proteins found within blood vessels. Matrix metalloproteinase–9 levels are significantly elevated in the white matter and **cerebrospinal fluid** (CSF) of patients with Binswanger type pathology. These increased levels of metalloproteinases in thickened penetrating arteries could promote leakage of fluid from these abnormal blood vessels. Chronic edema in perivascular areas could stimulate gliosis.

TREATMENT

This patient's blood pressure is too high, and all attempts should be made to lower it. Blood pressure should be monitored. Often it is helpful to use 24-hour ambulatory blood pressure monitoring. Nighttime blood pressure is very important. Nocturnal blood pressures that are too high or too low have been associated with clinical and brain imaging worsening. Since reducing whole blood viscosity can increase blood flow, reduction of hematocrits >45 (by blood donation and stopping smoking) and reducing fibrinogen levels by prescribing eicosapentaenoic-rich fish oil preparations should be considered. Liberalizing fluid intake is also important. Antiplatelets, especially extended release dipyridamole or cilostazole, are used because of their salutary effects on the vascular endothelium.

KEY POINTS TO REMEMBER

- There are 2 main types of vascular dementia: a) penetrating artery disease characterized by multiple lacunar infarcts and white matter loss and gliosis, and b) multiple cortical and/or subcortical infarcts caused by brain embolism or large artery occlusive disease or brain hemorrhages. The clinical **findings**, imaging, and treatment of these two groups are quite different.
- The penetrating artery type of vascular dementia (Binswanger disease) is most often caused by chronic hypertension, but polycythemia, CADASIL, and cerebral amyloid angiopathy can show similar findings.
- The most common findings in Binswanger patients are: pyramidal and extrapyramidal dysfunction, pseudobulbar dysarthria and dysphagia, abulia, slowness, and executive dysfunction.
- Brain imaging shows multiple basal ganglionic and thalamic and white matter lacunes and regions of white matter abnormalities with loss of white matter and compensatory hydrocephalus.
- Treatment includes control of hypertension, reduction in high hematocrits, liberal fluid intake, and antiplatelet agents.

Further Reading

Babikian V, Ropper AH. (1987). Binswanger disease: a review. *Stroke* 18:1-12.

Caplan LR. (1995). Binswanger's disease: revisited. *Neurology* 45:626-633.

Caplan LR, Schoene WC. (1978). Clinical features of subcortical arteriosclerotic encephalopathy (Binswanger's disease). *Neurology* 28:1206-1215.

Fisher CM. (1989). Binswanger's encephalopathy: a review. *J Neurol* 236:65-79.

Rosenberg GA, Sullivan N, Esiri MM. (2001). White matter damage is associated with matrix metalloproteinases in vascular dementia. *Stroke* 32:1162-1168.

13 Subarachnoid Hemorrhage (SAH)

A 45-year-old woman presented to the emergency room with a severe headache of two days' duration. Her medical history is notable for migraine headaches, but this headache is different. She felt a "popping" on the left side of her head followed rapidly by excruciating headache and she vomited. She took eletriptan as she does for her migraines and, when this failed to relieve her symptoms, took ibuprofen 800mg and went to bed. Her headache persisted the next day when she noted new neck pain and stiffness. In spite of repeat doses of ibuprofen, her symptoms were unremitting, so the next day she sought medical attention.

Her medical history is otherwise notable for hypertension diagnosed two years ago. She has no allergies and takes lisinopril daily. Her mother and sister each have migraine headaches and her father has high blood pressure. The family history was otherwise unremarkable. She works as a teacher, drinks a glass of wine with dinner, and smokes 1/2 pack of cigarettes each day as she has for the last ten years.

In the emergency room, she was afebrile and hypertensive with blood pressure 153/88. Heart rate was regular at 80 bpm, and respirations were 20. She appeared anxious and was lying still in bed. She had head and neck pain with passive flexion of the head and hips. She was alert and oriented but distracted by her headache. She was able to provide a consistent history; speech was fluid, prosodic, and without dysarthria. The patient followed multistep commands but had difficulty naming "watch band" and "tie clip." Fundoscopic exam was normal. Pupils were symmetric and reactive. Her eyes moved conjugately, but the patient reported pain with lateral gaze. Visual fields were full. Smile was symmetric. Appendicular strength was intact. Reflexes were symmetric, plantar responses were flexor. There was no pronator drift. Sensation was intact, and she did not extinguish to double simultaneous stimulation. She had no dysmetria or dysdiadochokinesia. The patient walked without assistance, albeit with discomfort.

She had a noncontrast head CT, which showed no hemorrhage or stroke. Complete blood count, PT/INR, and aPTT were normal. Serum chemistries were notable for mild hyponatremia at 133mMol/L. She subsequently had a CSF analysis by lumbar puncture, revealing elevated protein at 90mg/dL, normal glucose. Cell counts were elevated with 8 polymorphonuclear cells and 258 erythrocytes in the first tube and 7 polymorpho-nuclear cells and 294 erythrocytes in the fourth tube collected. Xanthochromia was not present by visual inspection but was positive on spectrophotometric analysis.

She was given intravenous fluids, antihypertensive medications, and magnesium sulfate and admitted to the hospital. The subsequent day she had cerebral angiography, which showed a 4mm irregularly shaped aneurysm at the bifurcation of the superior and inferior divisions of the left middle cerebral artery. The aneurysm was successfully coiled. The remainder of her hospital course was uneventful and she was discharged home.

What do you do now?

The evaluation of headache in the emergency room can be challenging. Headache is a common presenting problem, and only a minority of patients with headache harbor malignant pathology. This is offset, however, by the sometimes subtle features of patients with subarachnoid hemorrhage (SAH), a malignant headache with a greater than 40% mortality rate. The clinical presentation of SAH is typified by the sudden onset of severe headache ("worst headache of life"). This is often associated with brief loss of consciousness or nausea and vomiting. If the bleeding is substantial, resultant mass effect can precipitate seizures or lateralizing weakness. Up to half of patients with headache from subarachnoid hemorrhage have mild or otherwise atypical signs and symptoms. This fact underscores the importance of careful evaluation of patients with headache.

Headaches that raise concern for SAH have aphoristically been categorized as "first, worst, or cursed." A new headache should raise suspicion for SAH. This has special bearing on the migraineur population: a new headache is classified as a migraine only after several similar episodes, so the first episode should be regarded with suspicion. Likewise, patients with migraines are often familiar with their headaches, so a report of a "different" type of headache may signify a different process. Likewise, any "worst headache of my life," insofar as it remains the classic symptom, requires evaluation for SAH. Finally, the "cursed" headache is the one associated with an abnormal neurologic exam and should similarly prompt thorough evaluation. The clinical diagnosis of SAH is further informed by epidemiologic factors and associated risks. Prevalence is highest in the 5th through 7th decade with slightly more women than men affected. Family or personal history of cerebral aneurysm, Ehlers-Danlos syndrome, or adult polycystic kidney disease are risk factors. Hypertension, tobacco, and heavy alcohol use have been associated with aneurysmal subarachnoid hemorrhage.

The diagnosis can be straightforward if pursued. After clinical evaluation, noncontrast head CT should be performed. If performed 12 to 24 hours after onset of symptoms, sensitivity is better than 95%. However, imaging can still miss small SAH, especially from a sentinel bleed. When performed more than 48 hours after symptom onset, the sensitivity drops to around 50%, as subarachnoid blood becomes isodense. If head CT is not diagnostic, lumbar puncture is indicated. Opening pressure is elevated (>250mm H_2O), protein is commonly elevated, glucose is normal, and red cells are often found. Because the needle can injure dural venules on its course to the subarachnoid space, red cells must be counted in sequential tubes. If the sequential erythrocyte count drops, blood may be "traumatic," from venules. However, cell counts may occasionally fall in sequential tube analysis in SAH. By contrast, if the erythrocyte count does not fall, the blood is from subarachnoid space and SAH is diagnosed. Sometimes with small sentinel SAH, erythrocytes are not found in the CSF sampled in the lumbar space. However, erythrocytes in the CSF are rapidly lysed and, even in small volumes, can be detected by looking for xanthochromia. This is assessed either by visual comparison with a water-containing tube or, preferably with digital spectrophotometry. These hemoglobin degradation products can be found as early as two hours after bleeding and persist two weeks or longer in CSF. Advanced imaging is sometimes used. MR imaging with T2*sequence can be as sensitive as early noncontrast head CT, but likewise is imperfect. More intriguing is the use of CT angiography (CTA) as a non-invasive way to assess vasculature and specifically look for the suspected aneurysm. This modality is gaining popularity, as resolution is approaching that of formal catheter-based angiography. However, it is less reliable for finding aneurysms smaller than 3 mm and, unlike lumbar puncture, cannot identify non-aneurysmal sources of SAH (e.g., perimesencephalic hemorrhage). Additionally, if SAH is suspected and CTA is nondiagnostic, catheter-based angiography is required, thus exposing the patient to dye load and radiation twice. Catheter-based angiography remains the "gold standard" to diagnose SAH. Its diagnostic role is mainly to identify the presence, location, size, and morphology of the suspected aneurysm, but may be used in occasional instances if head CT and lumbar puncture analysis are nondiagnostic.

KEY POINTS TO REMEMBER

- Thunderclap headache, headache with associated neurological signs should raise suspicion for subarachnoid hemorrhage.

- Sensitivity of noncontrast head CT in diagnosing SAH can be more than 95% 12–24 hours after a bleed but drops to 50% after two days.
- Lumbar puncture to assess for subarachnoid blood or xanthachromia is most sensitive from 12 hours to 2 weeks after bleeding.
- CT angiography and MR imaging can be useful non-invasive adjunctive modalities to diagnose SAH, but catheter-based angiography remains the gold standard for diagnosis.

Further Reading

Adams HP, Jergenson DD, Kassell NF, Sahs AL. (1980). Pitfalls in the recognition of subarachnoid hemorrhage. *JAMA* 244:794-796.

Bederson JB, Connolly ES, Batjer J, et al. (2009). Guidelines for the management of aneurysmal subarachnoid hemorrhage. *Stroke* 40:994-1025.

Chappell ET, Moure FC, Good MC. (2003). Comparison of computed tomographic angiography with digital subtraction angiography in the diagnosis of cerebral aneurysms: a meta-analysis. *Neurosurg* 52:624-631.

Edlow JA, Caplan LR. (2000). Avoiding pitfalls in the diagnosis of subarachnoid hemorrhage. *N Engl J Med* 342:29-36.

Kaibara T, Heros R. (2008). Aneurysms. In: *Uncommon Causes of Stroke*, 2nd edition, (Caplan LR, ed.), pp. 171-180. Cambridge UK, Cambridge University Press.

Sidman R, Connolly E, Lemke T. (1996). Subarachnoid hemorrhage diagnosis: lumbar puncture is still needed when the computed tomography scan is normal. *Acad Emerg Med* 3:827-831.

Sidman R, Spitalnic S, Demelis M, Durfey N, Jay G. (2005). Xanthochromia? By what method? A comparison of visual and spectrophotometric xanthochromia. *Ann Emerg Med* 46:51-55.

14 Lobar Hemorrhage in Cerebral Amyloid Angiopathy

An 82-year-old man is brought to the emergency room by his family because of a severe headache and complaint that he cannot see to the right. He was reported to be well early that morning. After breakfast, he developed an occipital headache. He noticed he could not see the right-hand side of the newspaper he was reading so he called to his wife. Previous medical history was significant for hypertension, atherosclerotic cardiovascular disease, a left hemiparesis secondary to a right lenticulostriate territory lacunar infarct, and hypothyroidism. He has no allergies and takes aspirin, lisinopril, and levothyroxine. He does not drink alcohol but has a 50 pack-year smoking history.

He was taken to the emergency room, where he was found to be alert and normally conversant. Blood pressure was normal and heart rate was 95. Medical exam was unremarkable. Neurological exam was notable for intact speech, naming, repetition, and writing. The patient could not read—even what he had just written. Fundoscopic exam was normal. Pupils were symmetric and reactive. Eyes moved conjugately. There was a dense right-sided visual field defect. Smile was symmetric. Appendicular strength was intact. Reflexes were symmetric, plantar responses were flexor. Sensation was intact, and he did not extinguish to double simultaneous stimulation. He had no dysmetria or dysdiadochokinesia. The patient could walk normally without assistance.

Head CT was performed and showed an acute 3x3.5x2.5cm left occipital **intracerebral hemorrhage** (ICH) and right internal capsule and left **frontal lobe cortical** hypodensities. Also noted were patchy areas of subtle hypodensity bilaterally adjacent to the lateral ventricles. CBC, PT/INR, and aPTT were normal. Serum chemistries were normal. EKG showed sinus rhythm. The patient was admitted. Brain MRI including T1 postgadolinium and T2* (GRE) imaging was performed and showed the left occipital (ICH). There was no associated enhancement, mild perilesional edema and, on T2* sequence imaging, a prior hemorrhage in the left frontocortical region and several scattered areas of microhemorrhages in the bilateral temporal and occipital lobes as well as in bilateral thalami.

The patient remained clinically stable, albeit with a persistent field cut. He was given counseling on smoking cessation. His aspirin was discontinued at admission but resumed one week later.

What do you do now?

ntraparenchymal hemorrhage accounts for 15% of strokes, affecting more than 30,000 patients each year in the United States. It can be a severe illness with a 30-day mortality up to 50% in some populations. ICH is most commonly due to hypertension, amyloid angiopathy, or hemorrhagic tumor. Other less common causes include venous sinus thrombosis, coagulopathy most often due to warfarin use, ruptured arteriovenous fistula or malformation and hemorrhagic transformation of an ischemic infarct.

Several aspects of acute management of ICH are shared across the various etiologies. Anticoagulation should be reversed, antiplatelets often discontinued, and significant elevation in blood pressure (above mean arterial pressure of 130 mmHg) should be treated. Evaluation for the cause of ICH should be pursued, as some aspects of treatment depend upon the cause.

Among elderly patients, cerebral amyloid angiopathy (CAA) is a very common cause of ICH. It is associated with deposition and aggregation of amyloid protein and presumed resultant vessel-wall fragility. CAA is a pathologic diagnosis, but a diagnosis is often made on clinical grounds. A history of cognitive impairment or dementia, perhaps related to amyloid protein aggregation or apoprotein E e2/e4 allele carrier state such as in Alzheimer's dementia is associated with CAA. ICH due to CAA is associated with advanced age. Hemorrhage is lobar in location with temporal lobe followed by occipital, parietal, then frontal lobes in relative frequency. Hemorrhage in CAA is commonly recurrent, often in the same lobe or adjacent to a site of prior hemorrhage. MR imaging, if done with T2* (GRE) sequencing, can show clinically and radiographically occult microhemorrhages, thought to represent hemosiderin deposition. Microhemorrhages are also seen in the basal ganglia, where they are thought to represent stigmata and consequence of hypertension. Microhemorrhages in the subcortical-cortical junction within lobar regions are more strongly associated with CAA. Figure 14.1 is a T2*weighted MRI that shows several small microhemorrhages and regions of abnormal white matter in a patient with CAA.

Patients with ICH due to CAA may present with large hemorrhages; this fact combined with the advanced age of the average patient accounts for

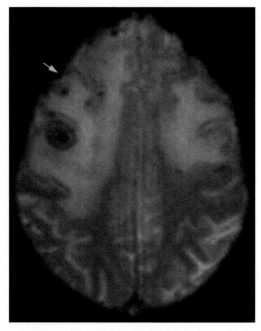

FIGURE 14.1   T2*weighted MRI showing small microhemorrhages in the upper left side of the scan (small white arrow) and regions of abnormal white matter in a patient with CAA.

much of the morbidity associated therein. However, ICH due to CAA may have a more favorable course with less predilection for edema formation and hemorrhage expansion. However, they portend significant risk for recurrence, as high as 20% over the subsequent two years. As such, a major management concern, particularly for patients with ICH due to CAA and confounding medical conditions is antithrombotic medication use. Because of the high risk for recurrence, anticoagulation is avoided. Likewise, antiplatelets such as aspirin, although less concerning than warfarin, will increase the risk of hemorrhage (with its attendant morbidity) by approximately 0.8%/year. As such, only patients with preexisting coronary artery disease or those with particularly high risk of stroke will likely benefit from resumption of antiplatelets after ICH due to CAA.

- CAA is a common cause of supratentorial lobar ICH.
- The differential diagnosis of spontaneous ICH includes CAA, hypertensive ICH, tumor, venous/sinus infarction, AVM, and hemorrhagic transformation of an ischemic infarct.
- CAA can be suggested by ICH without other apparent cause in patients age >55 and multiple hemorrhages in lobar regions.
- The presence of preexisting cognitive impairment, APOE e2 and e4 carrier status, or frank dementia may increase the likelihood of CAA diagnosis.
- CAA is often associated with hemispheric lobar microbleeds on T2* sequence MR imaging.

Further Reading

Cordonnier C, Leys D. (2008). Cerebral amyloid angiopathies. In *Uncommon Causes of Stroke*, 2nd edition (Caplan LR, ed.), pp. 455-464. Cambridge UK, Cambridge University Press.

Eckman MH, Rosand J, Knudsen KA, Singer DE, Greenberg SM. (2003). Can patients be anticoagulated after intracerebral hemorrhage? A decision analysis. *Stroke* 34(7):1710-1716.

Greenberg SM, Vonsattel JP, Segal AZ, et al. (1998). Association of apolipoprotein E epsilon 2 and vasculopathy in cerebral amyloid angiopathy. *Neurology* 50:961-964.

Massaro AR, Sacco RL, Mohr JP, et al. (1991). Clinical discriminators of lobar and deep hemorrhages: the Stroke Data Bank. *Neurology* 41:1881-1885.

Rosand J, Muzikansky A, Kumar A, et al. (2005). Spatial clustering of hemorrhages in probably cerebral amyloid angiopathy. *Ann Neurol* 58(3):459-462.

Smith EE, Gurol ME, Eng JA, et al. (2004). White matter lesions, cognition, and recurrent hemorrhage in lobar intracerebral hemorrhage. *Neurology* 63:1606-1612.

Vernooj MW, van der Lugt A, Ikram MA, et al. (2008). Prevalence and risk factors of cerebral microbleeds: the Rotterdam Scan Study. *Neurology* 70:1208-1214.

Dural Sinus Venous Thrombosis

A 32-year-old woman presented to the emergency room because she had had headache for three days. She had delivered her first child two weeks before presentation. Her pregnancy and delivery were uneventful, and she had no significant past medical history other than occasional headaches. She woke up three days ago with an intense generalized headache, that was mostly throbbing and worsened when she stood up. She had one episode of transient blurring of vision but no photo or phonophobia.

Her examination was normal with normal vital signs and no focal neurological deficits. She had CT scan of the head that was normal; a lumbar puncture showed an elevated opening pressure but otherwise normal CSF findings. An MRI/MRV showed thrombosis in the right transverse sinus and right jugular vein (Figure 15.1).

What do you do now?

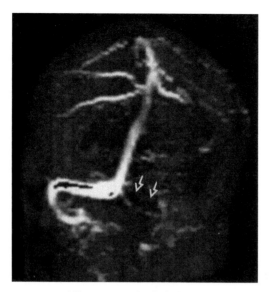

FIGURE 15.1 MR venogram. The straight sinus, deep veins, and lateral sinus are thrombosed and so are not seen on the right of the figure (white arrowheads point to the region of absent veins). From Caplan LR. (2009). Cerebral venous thrombosis. In: *Caplan's Stroke: A Clinical Approach*, 4th edition. Philadelphia, Saunders/Elsevier, with permission.

Headache during and after pregnancy is common and most often has a benign explanation. Nevertheless the diagnosis of primary headache disorders should be made only after thorough consideration of other diagnoses.

Migraine usually improves during pregnancy, and many women who have had an improvement of their migraine headaches will develop severe migraine headaches postpartum. This patient has some features consistent with migraine, yet the lack of previous similar episodes and the presence of postural visual changes raises red flags and warrant further work-up to exclude other causes.

Idiopathic intracranial hypertension (IIH) should be considered in young women with headache, visual obscurations, and high intracranial pressure with no mass lesion. IIH tends to worsen during pregnancy and may persist until early puerperium. It often occurs in obese women who gain weight rapidly during pregnancy. To diagnosis IIH one must exclude the presence of cerebral venous sinus thrombosis. Postural worsening of headache can be seen also in association with intracranial hypotension, which can occur as a complication of epidural anesthesia and CSF leak. In such cases, CSF pressure is low when measured.

Other differential diagnosis of severe acute headache in the puerperium include subarachnoid hemorrhage, reversible cerebral vasoconstriction syndrome (which includes postpartum cerebral angiopathy, eclampsia, and posterior reversible leukoencephalopathy syndrome), and pituitary apoplexy.

The diagnosis of cerebral venous sinus thrombosis (CVST) needs to be entertained in any patient with a peripartum headache, particularly if there is a change in headache quality, or if it is associated with focal neurological deficits. CVST remains an uncommon diagnosis in young women of childbearing age. The incidence is estimated to be about 10 per 100,000 deliveries, but it can lead to devastating disability and even death if not timely diagnosed and treated.

This condition has highly variable clinical presentations that range from headache with isolated intracranial hypertension to coma with severe neurological deficits. The most frequent presentation is with puerperal headache over several days. Usually it begins 1 day to 4 weeks postpartum and peaks in occurrence around 1–2 weeks postpartum.

Headache is present in 90% of CVST cases. It can be acute, subacute, or chronic. More often it is localized rather than diffuse. Other common features include focal neurological symptoms and signs, seizures, and altered consciousness and cognitive function.

The clinical presentation depends on the site and number of occluded sinuses and the presence of parenchymal brain lesions (such as cerebral edema, venous infarction, or hemorrhagic venous infarctions). For example, an isolated lateral sinus thrombosis often presents with isolated intracranial hypertension, and cavernous sinus thrombosis clinical presentation includes cranial neuropathy and other ocular findings; while in the case of deep venous sinus thromobosis (like straight sinus) this may produce impairment of consciousness and severe neurological deficits.

The etiology of CVST is divided into two large groups: septic and nonseptic. Nowadays in the era of antibiotics the former is uncommon and most cases are nonseptic. Several underlying conditions are associated with aseptic sinus thrombosis, including genetic or acquired prothrombotic conditions such as: pregnancy and the puerperium, malignancy, hematologic disorders, mechanical causes (head trauma, surgery, catheterization, and lumbar puncture), medications like oral contraceptives, hormonal replacement therapy, some chemotherapy agents, and dehydration. Often more than one underlying condition is present (most common pregnancy and hypercoaguable disorder) and in 15–25 % of cases there is no identified risk factor.

Inherited prothrombotic conditions associated with CVST include:

- activated protein-C resistance/factor V Leiden
- antithrombin III deficiency
- protein C or protein S deficiency
- antiphospholipid antibodies
- prothrombin gene mutation
- homocysteinemia (MTHFR mutation)

CVST is an elusive diagnosis because of its nonspecific presentation and its numerous predisposing causes. A high degree of suspicion is essential for rapid diagnosis. Radiological studies are crucial in establishing the definitive diagnosis. Computerized tomography "CT" scan of head is often the first imaging study obtained. It may show hyperdensity in the area of a thrombosed sinus or may show venous infarction or hemorrhage at the affected area. It is important to recognize that noncontrast enhanced CT can be normal in up to 50% of patients, which may falsely reassure the physician that there is no structural lesion. CT venography may show absence of contrast filling in the thrombosed sinuses. Magnetic resonance imaging (MRI) in combination with MR venography is the most often used imaging modality to diagnose CVST. The characteristics of the MRI signal depend on the age of the thrombus; this helps to determine the temporal onset of CVST. MRI is more sensitive than CT to show parenchymal brain lesions from venous infarctions, edema, or hemorrhage and MRV may show the absence of flow in the thrombosed sinuses. If MR studies are not diagnostic, conventional angiography should be considered especially if isolated cortical vein thrombosis is suspected.

Laboratory tests help show evidence of underlying thrombophilia, infection, or inflammation. D-dimer measurements can be used as a screening test for venous occlusive disease. D-dimer is a marker of endogenous fibrinolysis and is often detectable in patients with deep vein thrombosis. Plasma levels of D-dimer (fragments of cross-linked fibrin degraded by plasmin) have been shown to be sensitive for the diagnosis of deep vein thrombosis and pulmonary thromboembolism and are very often elevated in patients with CVST. CSF examination remains a useful diagnostic tool in CVT and should be performed after imaging to exclude brain abscess, massive cerebral hemorrhage, or infarction. Lumbar puncture is useful to remove CSF and reduce intracranial hypertension, as well as to exclude meningeal infections or carcinomatous meningitis as a cause for CVT.

Treatment, which is started as soon as the diagnosis is confirmed, consists of reversing the underlying cause when known and controlling seizures and intracranial hypertension; anticoagulation with IV heparin or low molecular weight heparin (LMWH) in acute phase followed by oral anticoagulation is indicated in nearly all patients with CVST even when there are parenchymatous hemorrhagic abnormalities on brain imaging. A few randomized controlled trails show that patient with venous sinus thrombosis appear to benefit from anticoagulation and appear to be safe. The duration of chronic anticoagulation is not firmly established and should be based on the underlying cause and the anatomical issue of recanalization. If a patient has an ongoing clotting disorder, they may benefit from long-term therapy. Local thrombolysis may be indicated in rare cases unresponsive to adequate anticoagulation especially when multiple dural sinuses are occluded.

The functional outcome after CVST is generally favorable with 60–86% of patients having complete recovery. CVST associated with pregnancy is relatively more benign than that occurring without it. History of previous CVST, older age than 30, and prior Caesarean section increase the risk of developing CVST during pregnancy. Factors that portend poor prognosis include focal deficits, encephalopathy and/or coma on presentation, presence of underlying infection or malignancy, and deep cerebral vein involvement.

KEY POINTS TO REMEMBER

- The onset of new headache during or after pregnancy should be considered an ominous sign until the secondary causes have been excluded.

- Headache most often precedes other symptoms and signs by days and even weeks.
- Most patients have elevated levels of D-dimer, which is a useful screening test.
- Brain and vascular imaging are critical for diagnosis. CT or MR venography or cerebral angiography can display the dural sinuses well.
- Early diagnosis and prompt treatment are essential to minimize morbidity and improve survival. Anticoagulation is the mainstay of acute and subacute treatment for CVST.

Further Reading

Bousser, M-G, Ferro JM. (2007). Cerebral venous thrombosis an update. *Lancet Neurol* 6:162-170.

Caplan LR. (2009). Cerebral venous thrombosis. In: *Caplan's Stroke: A Clinical Approach*, 4th edition, pp. 554-577. Philadelphia, Saunders/Elsevier.

Ferro JM, Canh,,o P. (2004). Stroke International Study on Cerebral Vein and Dural Sinus Thrombosis (ISCVT). *Stroke* 35:664-670.

Gladstone JP, Dodick DW, Evans R. (2005). The young woman with postpartum thunderclap headache. *Headache* 45:70-74.

Lanska DJ, Kryscio RJ. (2000). Risk factors for peripartum and postpartum stroke and intracranial venous thrombosis. *Stroke* 31:1274-1282.

Satm J. (2005). Thrombosis of the cerebral veins and sinuses. *N Engl J Med* 352:1791-1798.

Stam J, De Bruijn, DeVeber G. (2002). Anticoagulation for cerebral sinus thrombosis. *Cochrane Review* (4)CD 002005.

16 Reversible Cerebral Vasoconstriction Syndrome

A 32-year-old woman came to the emergency room of a hospital because that morning she had developed temporary numbness of her left hand and foot. She had delivered her third child 5 weeks before. The pregnancy was without event, as was the delivery. Her blood pressure was slightly high during the early postpartum days and weeks. Three weeks ago she had felt depressed and her physician prescribed sertraline to treat her depression and hydrochlorothiazide to control the blood pressure, which he measured at 150/85. Ten days ago she suddenly developed a very severe headache that quickly spread throughout her head. The headache abated after one hour, but similar less intense headache had been occurring daily since. She seldom was without some head discomfort. On one occasion she found it difficult to speak for several hours.

On examination, blood pressure 145/80, pulse 85 and regular. No neck or cranial bruits. Her neurological examination was normal except that she could not localize touch accurately in her left hand.

A CT examination showed a small area of superficial subarachnoid bleeding over the right paracentral convexity. An MRI confirmed the region of subarachnoid blood and also showed small areas of hyperintensity on FLAIR images in the lateral convexal portion of the right postcentral gyrus and the left frontal region. MRA and later cerebral dye contrast angiography showed regions of narrowing and dilatation involving the major large arterial branches of the intracranial arteries (Fig 16.1).

What do you do now?

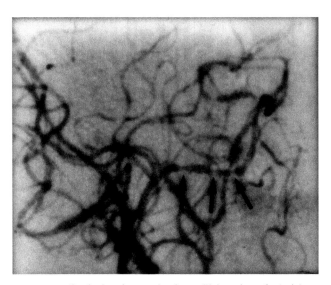

FIGURE 16.1 Cerebral angiogram showing multiple regions of arterial narrowing and dilatation producing "sausage shape" abnormalities.

This postpartum woman has developed a reversible vasoconstriction syndrome characterized by a "thunderclap" headache at onset, superficial subarachnoid bleeding, intracranial regions of vasoconstriction and vasodilatation, and small areas of brain ischemia.

French physicians had long been aware of a syndrome that they dubbed postpartum angiopathy. This entity was characterized by sudden onset of a severe headache sometime during the puerperium. Blood pressure was often high, and some women had accompanying findings that suggested preeclampsia (proteinuria, increased deep tendon reflexes, hyperactivity, and elevated blood pressure). Angiography in some of these patients showed regions of vasoconstriction.

Call, Fleming, and colleagues in 1988 called attention to a syndrome that they called reversible cerebral segmental vasoconstriction, which was not always related to pregnancy or the puerperium. Their patients' symptoms and angiographic evidence of vasoconstriction recovered often after weeks or a few months, as had the findings in patients with "postpartum angiopathy." These patients were variously treated with corticosteroids and other agents.

The advent of modern vascular imaging has made it clear that this syndrome of vasoconstriction is relatively common, and the condition is now most often referred to as the Reversible Cerebral Vasoconstriction Syndrome (RCVS). Some continue to use the designations "postpartum angiopathy" and "Call, Fleming syndrome." The usual symptoms, signs, and imaging findings have become well known, but there is still uncertainty about optimal treatment. Unfortunately the syndrome has not become sufficiently well known and recognized and is very often misdiagnosed as "vasculitis."

The RCVS syndrome most often affects young women, especially during the puerperium, but also occurs at menopause and is found at all ages. Many of the patients have had a history of migraine. Some patients have developed this syndrome after carotid endarterectomy. The use of serotonin reuptake inhibitors prescribed for depression, and cannabis especially smoked in a binge can provoke the syndrome. Drugs such as phenylpropanolamine, cocaine, and amphetamines can also precipitate identical syndromes.

The onset is very often with a so-called thunderclap severe headache. Recurrent headache, focal neurological symptoms and signs, and occasionally seizures are the predominant symptoms. Vasoconstriction involves many large, medium, and small-sized cerebral arteries. The clinical findings include severe headache, decreased alertness, seizures, and changing multi-focal neurological signs. Brain edema and death can occur but are not common. Brain imaging may show focal subarachnoid blood on the surface of the brain and in adjacent sulci and small regions of abnormality on FLAIR-MRI imaging representing small infarcts. Angiography shows sausage-shaped focal regions of vasodilatation and multifocal regions of vascular narrowing. Early vascular imaging, especially during the first week, may be normal. Vasoconstriction usually peaks between 14 and 21 days. Transcranial Doppler ultrasound (TCD) shows high velocities in many intracranial arteries. TCD can be frequently repeated and provides a good index of the extent of vasoconstriction. Some patients develop larger zones of brain edema, most often in the posterior portions of the cerebral hemispheres as part of a Posterior Reversible Encephalopathy Syndrome (case 17).

Corticosteroids, calcium channel blockers, anticonvulsants, and treatments for increased intracranial pressure have been used to treat this condition. My experience and that of others is that calcium-channel blockers that have effects on intracranial arteries (verapamil, nimodipine, and nicardipine) are quite effective, although the dose must be titrated. Serotonin reuptake inhibitors should be stopped. The blood pressure should be normalized, which is often the case with calcium-channel blockers without adding another agent.

Vasoconstriction syndromes are many times more common than true vasculitis, and the epidemiological, clinical, and imaging findings now should be well known. Although intracranial focal regions of arterial narrowing is a nonspecific sign, my experience is that radiologists and neuroradiologists continue to misdiagnose the findings as diagnostic of vasculitis. A chain of events ensues and rheumatologists (who know nothing about this neurological condition) are consulted and prescribe immunosuppressants and corticosteroids.

KEY POINTS TO REMEMBER

- Reversible Cerebral Vasoconstriction Syndromes (RCVS) are common, many times more common than vasculitis.
- Women are affected much more often than men, and the post-partum and early menopausal periods are frequent times of onset.

Use of serotonin reuptake inhibitors and drugs that affect catecholamine metabolism may trigger the syndrome.

- Onset is often abrupt with a so-called thunderclap severe headache, and headaches recur in the days and weeks after onset.
- Superficial regions of subarachnoid bleeding, and regions of brain infarction and brain edema occur and are well shown on brain imaging.
- Vascular imaging (CTA, MRA, dye contrast angiography) after the first week shows regions of alternating vasoconstriction and vasodilatation. Transcranial Doppler ultrasound shows a diffuse increase in intracranial blood flow velocities.
- Treatment with calcium-channel blockers, especially verapamil, nimodiopine, and nicardipine) is effective, but the dosage requires titration.

Further Reading

Call GK, Fleming MC, Sealfon S, et al. (1988). Reversible cerebral segmental vasoconstriction. *Stroke* 19:1159-1170.

Ducros A, Boukobza M, Porcher R, et al. (2007). The clinical and radiological spectrum of reversible cerebral vasoconstriction syndrome: a prospective series of 67 patients. *Brain* 130:3091-3101.

Ducros A, Bousser M-G. (2009). Reversible cerebral vasoconstriction syndrome. *Pract Neurol* 9:256-267.

Singhal AB, Bernstein RA. (2005). Postpartum angiopathy and other cerebral vasoconstriction syndromes. *Neurocrit care* 3:91-97.

Singhal AB, Koroshetz WJ, Caplan LR. (2008). Reversible cerebral vasoconstriction syndromes. In: *Uncommon Causes of Stroke*, 2nd edition (Caplan LR, ed.), pp. 505-514. Cambridge UK, Cambridge University Press.

17   Reversible Posterior Encephalopathy Syndrome

A 24-year-old recent college graduate was hospitalized because of hematuria. A neurological consultation was requested when he developed headache and loss of vision and had a grandmal seizure on the third hospital day.

About 8 days before admission he developed a sore throat and fever. Two days before hospitalization he noted dark urine almost the color of reddish ale. He had been previously well and had been on university sports teams. He now worked as a journalist. He had had no serious past illnesses. He had many girlfriends and had been sexually active with a number of partners, some of whom he picked up in bars. He never had taken cocaine or other drugs and did not drink excessively. His mother had systemic lupus erythematosis. His father had hypertension, well controlled with medications.

Examination on admission to the hospital had shown: pulse 72 and regular, blood pressure 165/95. He was alert but slightly lethargic. The recorded physical and scant neurological examinations were considered normal. His urine was red and contained red cell casts, white and epithelial cells, and a high protein content.

Blood urea nitrogen (BUN) was 60, and creatinine 3.5. The remainder of his blood tests showed no important abnormalities. Chest x-ray and head CT were normal on the day of admission.

On day 2 he complained of more severe headache and seemed relatively inattentive. Later that day he briefly thought that he saw animals and colored objects in his vision; later that day he said that he could not see. When tested he could not identify objects or colors although his pupils reacted well to light. His physicians consulted a psychiatrist to exclude a hysterical conversion reaction.

On the morning of the third hospital day he was more lethargic and his nurse witnessed a grand mal seizure. Examination by a neurologist showed that he was lethargic but could be aroused. His speech was spontaneously sparse but contained no paraphasic errors. His answers were brief but appropriate to the queries. He said he was in a hospital but could not recall the name or the day he was admitted. He was easily distracted and appeared restless and hyperactive. He could not recall any of the objects given to him to remember after 5 minutes. He claimed not to be able to see fingers or a necktie. Pupil size and reaction to light were normal, as was a careful view of his optic nerve and retina, and testing of cranial nerve functions. His limbs moved symmetrically. Deep tendon reflexes were brisk but symmetric. Plantar responses were flexor. An MRI scan showed bilateral parieto-occipital abnormalities on a FLAIR sequence (Fig 17.1).

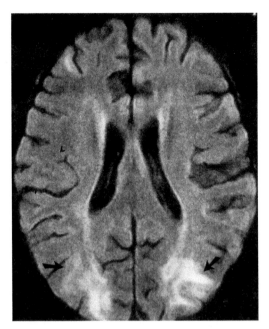

FIGURE 17.1 MRI FLAIR sequence showing bilateral parito-occipital abnormalities that spare the paramedian striate cortex.

Treatment of his blood pressure with diuretics and calcium-channel blockers was followed by rapid recovery of his neurological symptoms and signs and a return to normal of the brain imaging abnormalities. Kidney biopsy showed a presumably poststreptococcal acute glomerulonephritis.

What do you do now?

This patient had developed a syndrome that is now usually referred to as the Posterior Reversible Encephalopathy Syndrome (PRES). The advent of modern brain imaging has shown that the syndrome is relatively common and its precipitants and clinical and imaging features have now been well described. Many different conditions including preeclampsia and eclampsia are associated with the syndrome including: hypertensive encephalopathy, use of immunosuppressive drugs including cyclosporine and MK-506, pheochromocytoma, acute glomerulonephritis, and acute endocrinopathies. PRES can develop in some patients with incompletely treated Reversible Cerebral Vasoconstriction Syndromes, or RCVS (case 16).

The clinical findings are characterized by agitation and restlessness, confusion, seizures, and visual dysfunction that includes visual hallucinations and cortical blindness. Brain imaging most often shows white matter hyperintensities maximal in the occipital and posterior temporal white matter but sparing the paramedian occipital striate regions. This syndrome is likely a capillary leak syndrome related to endothelial dysfunction and increased body fluid volumes. In some patients the neurological abnormalities are accompanied by increased blood pressure, proteinuria, and tissue edema. Extensive experience has shown that the cortex as well as white matter are often involved, that the abnormalities can be frontal, brainstem, cerebellar, and diffuse and are not always limited to the posterior cerebral hemispheres. In some patients irreversible tissue damage develops, especially if the blood pressure elevations and edema are not treated rapidly and effectively.

The major differential diagnostic consideration in patients in whom the imaging abnormalities are limited to the posterior parieto-occipital regions is embolism to the bilateral posterior cerebral arteries causing brain infarction. The clinical setting, parietal (non-PCA territory) localization, and sparing of the striate calcarine cortex, and onset with seizures are findings that strongly favor PRES rather than embolism to the rostral basilar artery bifurcation.

KEY POINTS TO REMEMBER

- Brain edema most often localized in the posterior portions of the cerebral hemispheres develops in a variety of situations and is referred to as the Posterior Reversible Encephalopathy Syndrome (PRES).

- Common clinical settings include: preeclampsia and eclampsia are associated with the syndrome including: hypertensive encephalopathy, immunosuppressive drugs such as cyclosporine and MK-506, pheochromocytoma, acute glomerulonephritis, Reversible Cerebral Vasoconstriction Syndromes (RCVS), and acute endocrinopathies.
- The most common clinical findings are: agitation, hyperactivity, loss of vision, visual hallucinations, and seizures.
- Brain imaging shows regions of predominantly white matter edema, often localized to the posterior occipital-parietal regions but sparing the striate calcarine cortex.
- In some patients the brainstem and cerebellum are predominantly affected and sometimes the imaging abnormalities are more widespread and involve other cerebral lobes.

Further Reading

Digre K, Varner M, Caplan LR. (2008). Eclampsia and stroke during pregnancy and the puerperium. In: *Uncommon Causes of Stroke*, 2nd edition (Caplan LR, ed.). Cambridge, UK, Cambridge University Press 515–528.

Hinchey J, Chaves C, Appignani B, et al. (1996). A reversible posterior leukoencephalopathy syndrome. *N Engl J Med* 334:494–500.

Hinchey JA. (2008). Reversible leukoencephalopathy syndrome: what have we learned in the past 10 years? *Arch Neurol* 65:175–176.

Schwartz RB, Feske SK, Polak JF, et al. (2000). Preeclampsia-eclampsia: clinical and neuroradiographic correlates and insights into the pathogenesis of hypertensive encephalopathy. *Radiology* 217:371–376.

Singhal AB. (2004). Postpartum angiopathy with reversible posterior leukoencephalopathy. *Arch Neurol* 61:411–416.

18 Atrial Fibrillation–Related Brain Embolism

Patient MK is a 78-year-old right handed man with a history of atrial fibrillation on warfarin, hypertension, coronary heart disease, and congestive heart failure, who suddenly fell down on a golf course. His golf partner immediately came to his help and found him awake but completely unable to speak; the right side of his face was droopy, and his right arm was hanging limp by his side. The ambulance was immediately called, and the patient was brought to the nearest hospital.

In the emergency room, 35 minutes later, he was found to be afebrile with a blood pressure of 190/90 and a pulse rate in the 80s, irregular. He was awake but uttered no words and did not follow simple instructions. His pupils were 3 mm on the right and 2 mm on the left, reactive. Eyes were conjugately deviated to the left, but the examiner could move the eyes across the midline to the right with oculocephalic maneuvers. There was no blink to visual threat from the right although he consistently blinked on the left. Right face was droopy and he was unable to move the right arm or leg spontaneously or to noxious stimuli. The right toe was upgoing.

Laboratory results included normal blood counts, chemistries, and an **international normalized ratio** (INR) of 1.5. A noncontrast head CT scan was obtained that showed a hyperdense left middle cerebral artery (MCA), a sign consistent with a clot in the left MCA; there were no other early signs of ischemia or hemorrhage.

What do you do now?

A trial fibrillation (AF) is a very strong risk factor for stroke especially in the elderly. Presence of concomitant risk factors such as hypertension, prior stroke or transient ischemic attack (TIA), coronary artery disease, congestive heart failure, and diabetes significantly increase the risk of stroke from AF. Recently, scoring systems have been devised to reliably estimate risks of stroke in patients who have atrial fibrillation, such as the CHADS 2 scoring system, which is based on stroke risk factors. Echocardiography findings such as: an enlarged left atrium, a very low cardiac ejection fraction, spontaneous echo contrast, left ventricle akinesis or hypokinesis, left ventricular aneurysm, greatly increase the risk of cardiogenic embolism. Strokes due to AF tend to be large, are frequently debilitating, and carry an overall poor prognosis. Dose-adjusted warfarin has been shown in many studies to markedly reduce the risk of stroke in patients with AF. (Table 18.1.) Although, Mr. MK was taking warfarin on a regular basis, his INR levels were subtherapeutic. His last INR was checked 3 weeks ago and was mildly therapeutic, but his dose was not readjusted.

The current examination is diagnostic of a large left cerebral hemispheric dysfunction. Conjugate eye deviation is explained by involvement of frontal eye fields causing the eyes to deviate toward the ischemic hemisphere. The patient also has significant difficulty producing and understanding speech, implicating involvement of the language centers located in the parasylvian regions of the left cerebral hemisphere. Visual field abnormalities on the right may be due to interruption of the projecting optic radiation to the occipital lobe or from visual neglect from a parietal involvement. The pattern of weakness shows a severe and symmetrical involvement of the face, arm, and leg. Overall, the deficits correspond to a wide swath of brain territory supplied by the MCA. This corroborates with the findings on CT scan showing a thrombus in the left MCA stem occluding the origin of this artery.

One and a half hours have elapsed since the symptom onset when the results of all major investigations are back, and the treating neurologist is pondering her options. Systemic thrombolysis with intravenous recombinant tissue plasminogen activator (rt-PA) has been shown to be an effective treatment for acute ischemic stroke in large multicenter trials. The first randomized placebo controlled trial of rt-tPA conducted almost 12 years ago showed that systemic thrombolysis within three hours of the onset of

TABLE 18.1 Trials of Prophylactic Therapy in Patients with Atrial Fibrillation without Valvular Disease

Trial	Design	Results
Copenhagen AFASKA	1007 patients; mean age 73; Coumadin (INR 2.8–4.2) vs. Aspirin (75mg/day) vs. placebo	thromboemboli (stroke, TIA, systemic embolism) Coumadin 2%/year; Aspirin 5.5%/year; placebo 5.5%/year
BAATAF	628 patients; mean age 68; Coumadin (INR 1.5–2.7) vs. other medical Rx (could include Aspirin)	Coumadin 2 strokes (0.4%/year); Control 13 (3%/year). No benefit of Aspirin (8 of 13 strokes in controls on Aspirin); 2 hemorrhages–1 each group
SPAF	1330 patients; mean age 67; Warfarin-eligible patients randomized to Warfarin (INR 2-3.5), aspirin (325 mg/day), or placebo. Warfarin-ineligible patients randomized to aspirin or placebo.	Warfarin 2.3%/year vs. 7.4%/year placebo; stroke in Warfarin-ineligible Aspirin group 3.6%/year vs. 6.3% in placebo group. Major bleeding 1.5%, 1.4%, 1.6% in Warfarin, Aspirin, placebo groups.
EAFT	1007 patients; mean age 73; Warfarin-eligible patients randomized to Warfarin (INR 2.5-4), Aspirin (300 mg), or placebo. Warfarin-ineligible to Aspirin or placebo.	Strokes in 8% of 225 in Warfarin group, 15% of 404 in Aspirin group, 19% of 378 in placebo group. Major bleeding 2.8%/year Warfarin group and 0.9%/year Aspirin group.

(continued)

TABLE 18.1 (Continued) Trials of Prophylactic Therapy in Patients with Atrial Fibrillation without Valvular Disease

Trial	Design	Results
SPAF II	1100 patients; mean age 69.6; Warfarin (INR 2-4.5) vs. Aspirin (325 mg/day compared in patients <75 and patients >75	715 patients <75; ischemic stroke & systemic embolism 1.3%/year Warfarin vs. 1.9%/year Aspirin; major hemorrhage 0.9%/year Aspirin, 1.7%/year Warfarin; 385 >75; ischemic stroke & systemic embolism 3.6%/year Warfarin, 4.8%/year Aspirin; major bleeds 4.2% Warfarin*, 1.6% Aspirin
SPAF III	1044 patients with 1 or more risk factors; mean age 72; low-intensity fixed dose Warfarin (INR 1.2-1.5) plus Aspirin (325 mg/day vs adjusted dose Warfarin (INR 2-3)	INR 1.3 fixed dose Warfarin vs. INR target 2.4 adjusted group. Ischemic stroke & systemic embolism in 7.9% of fixed dose & Aspirin vs. 1.9% in adjusted dose group
	892 patients with posited low risk were given 325 mg Aspirin	The rate of ischemic stroke was low (2%/year) and disabling ischemic stroke only 0.8%/year. The rate of major bleeding was 0.5%/year
BAFTA	973 elderly (mean age 81.5) Warfarin (INR 2-3) vs. Aspirin 75mg/day	50% less of combined ischemic stroke, intracranial hemorrhage, systemic emboli in Warfarin group; annual risk of extracranial hemorrhage 1.4% Warfarin vs 1.6% aspirin

AFASAK–Copenhagen Atrial Fibrillation Aspirin Anticoagulation Study
BAATAF–Boston Area Anticoagulation Trial for Atrial Fibrillation
SPAF–Stroke Prevention in Atrial Fibrillation Study
EAFT–European Atrial Fibrillation Trial
■ 71% of intracranial hemorrhages fatal; 29% had residual deficit
From Caplan LR, *Caplan's Stroke: A Clinical Approach*, 4th edition, Philadelphia, Elsevier, 2008, with permission.

ischemic stroke improved clinical outcomes. More recently, the European Cooperative Stroke Study (ECASS) published the results of their randomized, placebo-controlled trial, showing that intravenous recombinant tissue plasminogen activator (IV rt-PA) was safe and effective in stroke patients between 3 to 4.5 hours after stroke onset. Both studies however, showed that t-PA was associated with an increased risk for intracerebral hemorrhage (ICH), which can be fatal. The treating physician has to weigh the risks and benefits of thrombolysis in this particular patient before making a final decision about therapy. She is aware that based on prior analysis, large stroke size, elevated blood pressure, high glucose levels, and coagulopathy increase the risk of ICH. Multimodal imaging such as diffusion/perfusion weighted brain MRI can provide reliable estimates of the extent of brain damage as well as penumbral tissues that are viable but at risk of infarction. However, in the absence of these imaging modalities, clinical examination and other clinical measures such as the NIH Stroke Scale (NIHSS) serves as a surrogate for estimating stroke size. Signs of early ischemia on a noncontrast head CT, such as loss of the gray-white differentiation in the cortical ribbon (particularly of the insula) or the lentiform nuclei and sulcal effacement are also associated with large infarction and poorer outcomes. The patient does not have any early signs of brain parenchymal injury but has a large stroke with an NIHSS of 22. MK also has severe hypertension, which increases the risk of brain hemorrhage with t-PA (a systolic blood pressure ≥185 mmHg or a diastolic blood pressure ≥110 mmHg is a contraindication to intravenous administration of rt-PA). The patient is mildly coagulopathic with an INR of 1.5 but below the cut-off level recommended for tPA (INR ≤ 1.7). The patient's neurologist decided to give him a dose of intravenous labetolol, which brought down his blood pressure to 164/84 mmHg. She concluded that the patient would benefit from tPA treatment after considering the overall risks and benefits and discussed these with the patient's wife. Mr. MK received a weight-based dose of rt-tPA 1 hour and 50 minutes after his neurological symptoms began. After spending 24 hours in the intensive care unit following thrombolytic treatment, his deficits improved significantly and he was now able to lift his right arm and leg off the bed and speak a few meaningful, short phrases. A repeat head CT showed a moderate sized deep and superficial MCA territory infarct without bleeding.

- Atrial fibrillation is a very important and common cause of brain embolism. Strokes from AF are often large and disabling.
- Standard anticoagulants have been shown in numerous trials to provide better prophylaxis against strokes in patients with non-valvular atrial fibrillation than placebo or antiplatelet agents.
- Decisions about using thrombolytic agents (either IV or IA) are often difficult and depend on many factors not only time from onset.
- The most important information that should guide treatment decisions about thrombolysis are: the location and size of brain infarction, the location and nature of any occlusive thromboemboli, and the amount of tissue at risk for further infarction.
- In each patient, the treating physician should weight the benefits and risks of all potential treatments and should share treatment decisions with the patient and responsible significant others whenever possible.

Further Reading

Albers G. (1994). Atrial fibrillation and stroke: three new studies, three remaining questions. *Arch Intern Med* 154:1443-1448.

Gage BF, Waterman AD, Shannon W, Boechler M, Rich MW, Radford MJ. (2001). Validation of clinical classification schemes for predicting stroke: results from the National Registry of Atrial Fibrillation. *JAMA* 285:2864-2870.

Hacke W, Kaste M, Bluhmki E, Brozman M, Davalos A, Guidetti D, Larrue V, Lees KR, Medeghri Z, Machnig T, Schneider D, von Kummer R, Wahlgren N, Toni D; for the ECASS Investigators. (2008). Thrombolysis with alteplase 3 to 4.5 hours after acute ischemic stroke. *N Engl J Med* 359:1317-1329.

Manning WJ. (2006). Cardiac source of embolism: treatment. In *Brain Embolism* (Caplan LR, Manning WJ, eds.), pp. 289-318. New York, Informa Healthcare.

The National Institute of Neurological Disorders and Stroke rt-PA Stroke Study Group. (1995). Tissue plasminogen activator for acute ischemic stroke. *N Engl J Med.* 333:1581-1587.

19 Management of the Patient with Acute Brain Ischemia

A 68-year-old woman presented with sudden onset of right sided weakness and impaired speech. She is known to have hypertension controlled on a single antihypertensive agent. She arrived at the emergency department 4 hours and 20 minutes after symptom onset. She was examined immediately and noted to have an irregular heart rate of 105, blood pressure 175/85. Her head and eyes were deviated to the left; she had a global aphasia, right hemiplegia involving the face and arm more than leg, and she did not blink to threat during visual stimuli presented from the right. Her National institute of health stroke scale (NIHSS) was 18.

A CT scan of the brain showed no intracranial hemorrhage. There were subtle early ischemic changes including loss of the left insular ribbon gray-white matter differentiation and obscuration of the lentiform ·nucleus.

CT angiography/CT perfusion showed occlusion of the proximal (M1) left middle cerebral artery (MCA) and a sizable penumbra. Complete blood count, chemistry, and coagulation laboratory results were normal.

Electrocardiogram (EKG) showed atrial fibrillation and no ST changes.

She is now 5 hrs from symptoms onset.

What do you do now?

A focused history, physical examination, and a CT scan are sufficient in this patient not only to exclude acute ischemic stroke mimics but also to identify the vascular lesion and the stroke mechanism that will eventually guide therapy.

In this case, clinical deficits and radiological findings are all consistent with left middle cerebral artery ischemia, and the most likely mechanism is cardioembolism in the setting of atrial fibrillation. Treatment options to consider are: 1) medical treatment with antithrombotic agents and maximization of blood pressure and blood volume to optimize collateral perfusion, 2) intravenous t-PA, 3) intra-arterial t-PA infused through an endovascular approach, and 4) mechanical thrombectomy with or without use of tPA or a GpIIb/IIIa inhibitor.

Occlusion of the mainstem MCA carried a poor prognostic outlook with a large area of decreased perfusion. The outlook to recover from this dominant hemisphere stroke without recanalization of the MCA (either spontaneously or iatrogenically) was poor. Medical treatment was plausible but not likely to be very effective. Adminstration of tissue-type plasminogen activator intravenously (IV tPA) would necessitate a larger infusion than if given directly into the thrombus and would have a high risk of bleeding. Use would also be outside the intravenous thrombolytic time window. Endovascular therapy using intra-arterial tPA and/or mechanical thrombectomy seemed to us to offer the best chance for adequate reperfusion of the presently ischemic zone, which was quite large and theoretically salvageable. The embolus wedged into the MCA should be easier to lyse or remove than an in-situ organized thrombus.

The risks and benefits of intra-arterial therapy and the other potential therapeutic strategies were discussed thoroughly with the family, and the decision was made to proceed with endovascular treatment. The patient was taken to the interventional suite, and her cerebral angiogram confirmed a complete occlusion of the proximal left MCA (Fig 19.1a). Successful recanalization was achieved through a combination of intra-arterial tPA and mechanical clot disruption and restoration of blood flow was observed in the MCA (Fig 19.1b) and left hemisphere of the brain after the intervention.

The patient was found to have improvement in her neurological examination 24 hours after the procedure. She was able to follow some commands

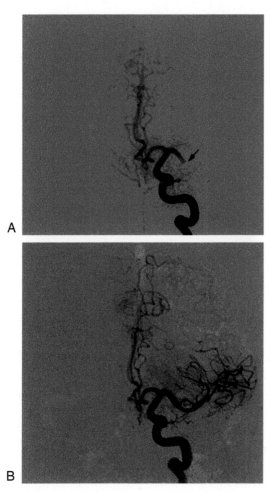

FIGURE 19.1 a. Cerebral angiogram showing occluded MCA (small black arrow).
b. Cerebral angiogram after thrombolysis showing recanalization and open MCA.

and move her right arm against gravity. Following a short hospitalization, she was discharged to a rehabilitation facility after initiation of secondary prevention measures. She made a good recovery and was able to manage independently at home months after her stroke.

Until recently, the only treatment available for stroke was prevention. The availability of effective treatment that could alter outcome within the first hours after stroke onset dramatically changed the care of acute stroke patients. Every patient with potentially acute brain ischemia was now considered as an eminently treatable neurological emergency.

The rationale for acute stroke treatment is based upon the concepts of the ischemic penumbra that represents tissue that is functionally impaired but structurally intact. Salvaging this tissue by restoring its normal blood flow is the aim of reperfusion therapy. The window for such therapy is brief, and in most patients this threatened tissue is no longer salvageable much beyond 8 hours after symptom onset.

The decision on thrombolytics depends on the presence and extent of brain infarction and the presence, location, and nature of arterial occlusion. No thrombolytics are given if the infarct is large and/or there is no arterial occlusion shown. Magnetic resonance studies including MRA, diffusion-weighted imaging (DWI), and perfusion-weighted imaging) (PWI) can yield information about the extyent of brain already infarcted, the presence and location of arterial occlusion, and the region that is underperfused but not yet infracted (the penumbra) (Fig 19.2). Thrombolytics are given if there is substantial at-risk brain tissue and a large intracranial artery occlusion. The selection of IV vs. IA thrombolytics depends on the location of the arterial occlusion, time since onset, and the availability of an experienced interventionalist. Systemic thrombolytics should be avoided if the patient is at high risk for systemic or brain hemorrhage.

The only therapy now approved for acute stroke by the U.S. Food and Drug Administration (FDA) and the European Union is intravenous tPA. This treatment should be administered to eligible patients who can be treated within 3 hours from onset of symptoms. Recent studies have provided new data on intravenous tPA treatment in the 3-to-4.5–hour window in carefully selected patients. But what if the patient is being treated at a time more than 4.5 hours after symptoms of brain ischemia began? Doctors owe it to their patients to consider all potential treatments and their benefits and risks in regard to the situation in the individual patient who is being treated. Some of the potential treatments may not be fully approved but still can be used with the acceptance and knowledge of the patient and their significant others.

Where adequate facilities and expertise are available, emergency angiography allows for mechanical clot removal and delivery of intra-arterial

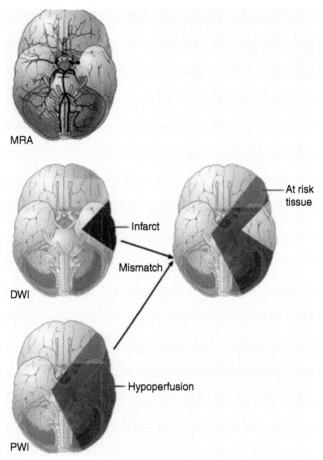

MRA

At risk tissue

Infarct

Mismatch

DWI

Hypoperfusion

PWI

FIGURE 19.2 Cartoon showing MRI evaluation of acute stroke patient. From *Caplan's Stroke: A Clinical Approach*, 4th edition, Philadelphia, Elsevier, 2009, with permission.

DWI=diffusion-weighted image

PWI=Perfusion-weighted image

MRA=Magnetic resonance angiogram

thrombolytic agents. Such therapies have been shown to promote early recanalization and some clinical benefit when applied within 6 hours of symptoms onset. In selected patients benefit also has been noted even after 24 hours. Intra-arterial thrombolysis potentially represents a means of overcoming some of the limitations of intravenous thrombolysis, which allows an increase in the number of patients eligible for thrombolytic therapy.

Therapy for acute stroke includes much more than thrombolysis. Appropriate management of blood pressure, glucose, intravenous fluids, temperature, and admission to stroke units all contribute to the overall outcome from acute stroke. Patients presenting with acute brain ischemia should have a thorough evaluation that includes: a history of the present events and risk factors, a quick targeted examination, and vascular imaging (including either a CT scan with CTA and CT perfusion imaging or MRI with DWI, T2* weighted imaging, MRA, and MR perfusion), cardiac tests, and basic laboratory evaluation.

Acute ischemic stroke care is a rapidly evolving field, and many ongoing trials are investigating new generation thrombolytics such as desmoteplase and tenecteplace (TNK), use of adjunctive therapies such as transcranial ultrasound and GPIIb/IIIa platelet receptor blockers. Other emerging therapies and strategies that are under investigation include novel catheter-based devices to enhance recanalization, utility of combination of IV-IA therapy, augmenting blood flow, neuroprotection, and imaging-based selection for recanalization treatment beyond the convential time window.

Stroke remains a leading cause of death and disability. All measures used to reduce mortality and disabilities are an important contribution to health care. Actions taken in the first few hours of stroke will determine the quality of patients' existences for the rest of their lives.

KEY POINTS TO REMEMBER

- Every patient who presents with acute brain ischemia should be viewed as an eminently treatable neurological emergency.
- The goals of initial evaluation are to confirm diagnosis of brain ischemia, exclude mimics, and identify the vascular lesion and stroke mechanism.
- Patients presenting with acute brain ischemia should have a thorough evaluation that includes: a history of the present events and risk factors, a quick targeted examination, and brain and vascular imaging (including either a CT scan with CTA and CT

perfusion imaging or MRI with DWI, T2*weighted imaging, MRA, and MR perfusion).

- Time window for effective therapy in stroke is brief. "Time is brain": The sooner the treatment is initiated after ischemic stroke, the more likely it is to be beneficial. All potential treatments and their relative benefits and risks should be considered.
- The decision on thrombolytics depends on the presence and extent of brain infarction and the presence, location, and nature of arterial occlusion. No thrombolytics are given if the infarct is large and/or there is no arterial occlusion shown.
- Appropriate management of blood pressure, glucose, intravenous fluids, temperature, and admission to stroke units all contribute to the overall outcome from acute stroke.

Further Reading

Adams HP Jr, del Zoppo G, Alberts MJ, et al. (2007). Guidelines for the early management of adults with ischemic stroke: AHA/ASA guidelines. *Stroke* 38:1655-1711.

Albers GW, Amarenco P, Easton JD, et al. (2008). Antithrombotic and thrombolytic therapy for ischemic stroke: ACCP Evidence-Based Clinical Practice Guidelines (Eighth Edition). *Chest* 133:630S-669S.

Caplan LR. (2009). *Caplan's Stroke: A Clinical Approach*, 4th edition. Boston, Butterworth-Heinemann, pp. 146-217.

Del Zoppo GJ, Saver JL, Jauch EC, Adams HP Jr. (2009). Expansion of the time window for treatment of acute ischemic stroke with intravenous tissue plasminogen activator: a science advisory from the American Heart Association/American Stroke Association. *Stroke* 40:2945-2948.

Hacke W, Kaste M, Bluhmki E, et al. (2008). Thrombolysis with alteplase 3 to 4.5 hours after acute ischemic stroke. *N Engl J Med* 359:1317-1329.

Lyden P (ed.). (2005). *Thrombolytic Therapy for Acute Stroke*, 2nd edition. Totowa, NJ, Humana press, pp. 211-234.

Meyers PM, Schumacher HC, Higashida RT, et al. (2009). Indications for the performance of intracranial endovascular neurointerventional procedures: a scientific statement from AHA/ASA. *Circulation* 119: 2235-2249.

20 Patent Foramen Ovale– Paradoxical Embolism

A 42-year-old man was brought to the clinic by a young woman. He said that after awakening in the morning, he had fallen as he went to the bathroom and found that his left limbs were weak and tingly. Since then he had improved, but his left cheek and hand still felt numb. The woman said that she had gone to sleep early while he sat on his knees on the bed drinking beer and watching a movie on television. He had awakened her at about 2 AM and had begun intercourse. During sex, his body had gone limp, and he was temporarily unarousable. She went to the kitchen to drink water and when she returned he was asleep.

He had no vascular risk factors but had injured his right leg 10 days ago.

There were no cardiac or vascular abnormalities on examination. His right calf was swollen and bruised. Cranial nerve examination including visual fields was normal except for slight flattening of the left nasolabial fold. His limbs were strong, but he could not localize touch well on the fingers of his left hand. His left biceps and brachial reflexes were brisker than the right. His left plantar response was extensor.

Blood studies were normal. A CT scan suggested a small right paracentral infarct. A CTA was normal. A transthoracic echocardiogram was normal but a transesophageal study showed a patent foramen ovale with bowing and abnormal mobility of the atrial septum (an atrial septal aneurysm). Doppler studies showed an occlusion of deep veins in his right leg.

What do you do now?

This patient had had a paradoxical embolus pass through a patent foramen ovale to reach the lateral paracentral portion of his right cerebral cortex. The thrombus likely originated in his right leg.

By far the most common potential intracardiac shunt is a patent foramen ovale (PFO). The interatrial septum begins to form early during uterine life. The septum primum grows caudally from the superior portion of the single atrium and fuses with the endocardial cushion closing the defect called the ostium primum. Another potential defect forms from partial resorption of the septum primum and is called the ostium secundum. A second septum, the septum secundum, arises from the superior portion of the atrium and descends on the right side of the septum primum to cover the ostium secundum. The ostium secundum is not covered completely because of the presence of the foramen ovale. The foramen ovale consists of the septum primum and septum secundum, which are joined parallel to a slitlike valve. This valve allows oxygenated blood to bypass the pulmonary circulation of the fetus during intrauterine life. At necropsy among individuals in the first 3 decades of life about a third have a PFO; the frequency decreases to 25% during the 4th–8th decades, and 20% during the 9th and 10th decades. The average diameter of PFOs is 4.9mm, and the size tends to increase with age. Paradoxical embolism has also been described through ventricular septal defects, atrial septal defects, and pulmonary arteriovenous fistulas.

The high frequency of PFOs among normal adults has made it important in an individual stroke patient to judge whether paradoxical embolism through the PFO was the cause of their stroke or whether the PFO was merely an incidental finding. I apply 5 criteria to judge the likelihood of a PFO as the source of brain embolism: 1) a situation that promotes thrombosis of leg or pelvic veins e.g., long sitting in one position, recent surgery, etc.; 2) increased coagulability, e.g., the use of oral contraceptives, presence of factor V Leiden with resistance to activated protein C, dehydration; 3) the sudden onset of stroke during sexual intercourse, straining during bowel movements, coughing, or other activity that includes a Valsalva maneuver or that promotes right-to-left shunting of blood; 4) pulmonary embolism within a short time before or after the neurological ischemic event; and 5) the absence of other putative causes of stroke after thorough evaluation. Echocardiographic features that increase the likelihood of embolism through a PFO are: atrial septal aneuryms, a large size, spontaneous passage of bubbles without necessitating a Valsalva maneuver, a large number of bubbles that pass through, and rarely a thrombus seen during echocardiography traversing the foramen ovale. In this patient the injured leg and prolonged sitting on the leg provided a suitable source of a thrombus and sex provoked the embolism. He had no competing potential causes. The most common territory of stroke is the middle cerebral artery (MCA), but the vertebrobasilar territory is involved more than explained by chance.

TREATMENT

Treatment options for patients with stroke and a patent foramen ovale include medical therapy with anticoagulants or antiplatelet agents, percutaneous closure using various devices, and direct surgical closure. Clearly patients with a PFO should be educated to avoid situations that promote thrombosis including prolonged sitting postures that promote venous stasis and thrombosis (such as a long vehicle ride, dehydration, oral contraceptives, etc.). Recurrence of paradoxical embolism is low even in the absence of antithrombotic therapy. Studies show a frequency of about 2–3% recurrence rate with either antiplatelet or anticoagulant prophylaxis. The rate of recurrence is slightly higher in the presence of an atrial septal aneurysm.

I suggest reviewing the treatment alternatives with this patient. Antiplatelet agents are effective and easy to use and the complication rates are low. Aspirin is probably as effective as other antiplatelets. Warfarin anticoagulation is more difficult to control at an optimal **international normalized ratio** (INR) level and requires frequent blood monitoring. Newer anticoagulants are available that are safer than warfarin and require less monitoring. The presence of an atrial septal aneurysm in addition to his PFO confers a bit higher risk and anticoagulation with either warfarin or dabigatran would probably provide more protection from recurrence than antiplatelets but also carries a higher bleeding risk. I also suggest reviewing the potential surgical and device alternatives. Open surgery as the initial treatment is seldom warranted unless medical treatment fails. Newer and more user-friendly and effective devices are still being developed and there is a learning curve for their safe introduction. I refer patients who want more information to a cardiologist who has had experience and success in implanting devices in order for the patient to learn of the potential risks and benefit of device implantation.

KEY POINTS TO REMEMBER

- Paradoxical embolism, arising from thrombi that arise in the leg or pelvic veins, and passing through a patent foramen ovale to reach the left ventricle of the heart, and subsequently the brain, has become an increasingly important cause of stroke.
- Diagnostic problems arise because as many as 25-30% of individuals have a PFO, and this common cardiac finding is often unrelated to the cause of the patient's brain ischemia.
- I apply five criteria that favor identification of the PFO as the source of brain embolism: a) a situation that promotes thrombosis of leg or pelvic veins; b) increased coagulability; c) the sudden onset of stroke during sexual intercourse, straining during bowel movements, coughing, or other activity that includes a Valsalva maneuver or that promotes right-to-left shunting of blood; d) pulmonary embolism; and e) the absence of other putative causes of stroke after thorough evaluation.
- A large foramen, spontaneous passage of injected bubbles, and a large shunt favor paradoxical embolism as an etiology of brain ischemia.
- Treatments include antiplatelets, anticoagulants, percutaneous closure devices, and open cardiac surgery repair.

Further Reading

Caplan LR, Manning WJ. (2006). Cardiac sources of embolism: the usual suspects. In: *Brain Embolism* (Caplan LR, Manning WJ, eds.), pp. 129-159. New York, Informa Healthcare.

Cramer S, Rordorf G, Maki J, et al. (2004). Increased pelvic vein thrombi in cryptogenic stroke: results of the Paradoxical Emboli from Large veins in Ischemic Stroke (PELVIS) study. *Stroke* 35:46-50.

Dastur CK, Cramer SC. (2008). Paradoxical embolism and stroke. In: *Uncommon Causes of Stroke*, 2nd edition (Caplan LR, ed.), pp. 483-490. Cambridge UK, Cambridge University Press.

Mas J-L, Arquizan C, Lamy C, et al. (2001). Recurrent cerebrovascular events
     associated with patent foramen ovale, atrial septal aneurysm, or both. *N Engl J Med*
     345:1740–1746.
Manning WJ. Cardiac sources of embolism: pathophysiology and identification. In:
     Brain Embolism (Caplan LR, Manning WJ, eds.), pp. 161–186. New York,
     Informa Healthcare.

Arterial Dolichoectasia with Pontine Infarction

A 75-year-old man presented to an emergency department at noon reporting right-sided hemiparesis and dysarthria. One week before, he had a transient episode of right face, arm, and leg weakness, and dysarthria lasting thirty minutes with complete resolution. On the day of presentation, he awoke at 7 AM with similar symptoms but they persisted. For about a year he had had daily, brief, left-sided lancinating facial pains that were excruciating. This facial pain was triggered and exacerbated by chewing or touching the left side of his face. His past medical history was significant for hypertension, hyperlipidemia, and cigarette smoking (30 pack-years). His medications included hydrochlorothiazide 25mg daily and simvastatin 20mg qhs. He was not taking antiplatelet medication.

On examination, his blood pressure was 160/92, pulse was 76 and regular. No carotid or vertebral bruits were auscultated. No arrhythmia or murmur was noted. Neurological examination was notable for moderate dysarthria, hypersensitivity to touch and pinprick in the left V2 region of his face, right lower facial droop, and severe weakness of the right arm and leg in an upper motor neuron distribution.

Noncontrast brain CT did not show an infarct or hemorrhage. MRI of the brain showed an acute small infarct involving the left pontine base on diffusion-weighted imaging. MRA of the brain and neck without contrast showed an ectatic basilar artery that deviated to the left and compressed the left trigeminal nerve. The mid-basilar artery was 30% stenosed. Transthoracic echocardiogram did not show a cardioembolic source. Telemetry did not reveal any arrythmias. Fasting lipid panel revealed total cholesterol 220 mg/dl, LDL 160 mg/dl, triglycerides 250 mg/dl, and HDL 40 mg/dl. The patient was started on aspirin 325mg daily and simvastatin was increased to 80mg qhs. For the trigeminal neuralgia, he was given trileptal 150 mg bid that was increased to 300 mg bid two weeks later.

What do you do now?

This patient has a dolichoectatic basilar artery with mid-basilar atherosclerotic disease. Most likely, a thrombus formed that temporarily occluded the origin of a left pontine branch artery causing the initial transient ischemic attack. One week later, the branch artery became completely occluded, resulting in the small left anterior pontine artery infarct. The dolichoectatic vessel was also compressing the left trigeminal nerve, resulting in trigeminal neuralgia.

Dolichoectasia refers to dilated and tortuous arteries; posterior circulation arteries are more often affected than in the anterior circulation. Increasingly, dolichoectasia is called "dilatative arteriopathy" because dilatation appears to be the most significant abnormality. No consensus has yet been established regarding the vessel diameter that is considered dolichoectatic. Incidence estimates of dolichoectasia range from 0.06 to 5.8%. Dolichoectatic vessels can be due to atherosclerosis, congenital causes, or dissection. Atherosclerotic dolichoectasia occurs most often in patients older than 40, especially men, and tends to affect the intracranial vertebral and basilar arteries. Congenital dolichoectasia typically affects patients younger than 40, especially woman. Distal branches of cerebral arteries and the posterior cerebral arteries are more often affected by congenital dolichoectasia. Diseases that may predispose to congenital dolichoectasia include Marfan's syndrome, Ehlers-Danlos syndrome, AIDS, Fabry's disease, sickle cell anemia, and alpha-glucosidase deficiency. Patients with congenital dolichoectasia may also develop superimposed atherosclerosis.

Other vascular malformations bear similarities to dolichoectasia. Fusiform aneurysms are ectatic vessels with a focal aneurysmal outpouching. Large fusiform aneurysms are referred to as giant serpentine aneurysms.

Multiple clinical manifestations of dolichoectasia include ischemic stroke, hemorrhagic stroke, compression of cranial nerves and the brainstem, and hydrocephalus. Compression of cranial nerves may cause hemifacial spasm, trigeminal neuralgia, diplopia, dysarthria, dysphagia, tinnitus, and vertigo, among others. Pontine or medullary compression often leads to ataxia, vestibular deficits, and weakness, including quadriparesis. Patients may have intermittent vestibulocerebellar symptoms for years prior to a stroke.

Dolichoectasia can predispose to stroke via several mechanisms. Ectatic vessels often have abnormal blood flow with sharply decreased blood flow velocities. Flow can be turgid and can even reverse direction. Decreased blood flow can result in thrombus formation. Atherosclerotic plaques, sometimes with calcification, may protrude into the arterial lumen and facilitate thrombus formation. Thrombi may block the lumen of branch arteries or embolize distally. Elongated and tortuous arteries may distort the orifices of branch arteries, especially in the pons, thereby decreasing flow and causing infarcts. One study of 29 patients with dolichoectatic basilar arteries found that 2/3 of patients had pontine infarcts. Fifty percent of the patients in the study also had thalamic, midbrain, and PCA territory infarcts.

Fragile dolichoectatic arteries may rupture and cause subarachnoid hemorrhage or intracranial hemorrhage. This fragility may be due to defects in the internal elastic lamina, or smooth muscle atrophy causing irregular thickness of the media. Fibrosis of the artery may be present. Risk factors for intracranial bleeding include hypertension, the basilar artery's lateral displacement and maximum diameter, use of antiplatelet or anticoagulant medications, and female gender.

Risk factors and type of ischemic disease associated with dolichoectasia were assessed by an epidemiological study called GENIC (Étude du Profil Génétique de l'Infarctus Cerebral). This study of 466 patients found that older age, male sex, hypertension, history of myocardial infarction, and increased thoracic aortic arch diameter are risk factors. Also, small vessel ischemic disease including multilacunar infarcts, leukoaraiosis, and *état criblé* (dilated Virchow-Robbins spaces around penetrating arteries) was prevalent. The GENIC study suggests that dolichoectasia is not only a systemic disease of large arteries, but also a disease of microscopic-sized arteries.

The optimal non-invasive imaging modalities for dolichoectasia are CTA or MRA with contrast. These tests enable characterization of the ectatic vessel's diameter and lateral displacement, and thrombus location. Transcranial Doppler ultrasound shows flow velocity within the dolichoectatic vessel and any reversal of flow. Conventional dye contrast angiography provides the best resolution of vessels, including smaller vessels branching off from the dolichoectatic section, and intramural thrombi. It gives valuable information about the direction and turbulence of flow. Of note, the radiological appearance of dolichoectasia (i.e., degree of cranial nerve or brainstem compression) does not always correlate well with the degree of clinical deficit.

The prognosis for patients with dolichoectasia is highly variable, ranging from benign to malignant. In one study, dolichoectasia progressed in 43% of patients, and occurred more frequently in younger patients and those with anterior circulation involvement. Overall, there is a high frequency of recurrent events. One study of 93 patients over 11 years found that 60% had at least one clinical event, of which ischemic strokes comprised 80%. A longitudinal study of 156 patients with vertebrobasilar dolichoectasia found an elevated risk of intracranial hemorrhage. The subarachnoid incidence was 2.2 per 1,000 person-years. The intracerebral hemorrhage incidence was 11.0 per 1,000 person-years. In contrast, population-based studies have shown a subarachnoid hemorrhage incidence of 0.06–0.09 events per 1,000 person-years, and an intracerebral hemorrhage incidence of 0.24–0.48 per 1,000 person-years. Patients have a higher recurrence risk of ischemic rather than hemorrhagic strokes.

Treatment of dolichoectasia remains uncertain. Antiplatelet or anticoagulant treatments have limited effectiveness, perhaps due to multiple stroke mechanisms other than atherosclerosis. In one prospective study, patients who initially presented with ischemia or other symptoms due to vertebrobasilar dolichoectasia and who were treated with antiplatelets or anticoagulants had a higher incidence of hemorrhage. Further study is needed to assess the risks and benefits of antiplatelet or anticoagulation treatment for vertebrobasilar dolichoectasia. Caution is advised in giving antiplatelets or anticoagulants to vertebrobasilar dolichoectasia patients who present with symptoms other than ischemia (e.g., hemifacial spasm or cranial nerve deficits).

Whether to pursue surgical treatment of dolichoectatic arteries and fusiform aneurysms is often unclear, and the intervention itself can be challenging. Unlike saccular aneurysms, these vessels lack a definable neck that can be surgically clipped while still preserving the parent vessel. Surgical intervention may cause bleeding or may compromise the distal blood supply. Some surgical options include trapping with bypass, proximal occlusion, resection with anastomosis, and transposition. Outcomes in a study of 40 patients at 3 years who underwent a variety of surgical treatments were good, with 78% of patients having Glasgow Outcome Scale scores of 1.

Anterior circulation interventions had superior outcomes than posterior circulation interventions (90% versus 65%). There were no perioperative deaths in the series, but 30% of patients had complications including hematomas, parent vessel thrombosis, or new cranial nerve deficits. More research is needed to determine which patient should undergo surgical intervention and which intervention is optimal.

KEY POINTS TO REMEMBER

- Dolichoectatic vessels may be congenital or atherosclerotic. Atherosclerosis may be engrafted upon congenital forms.
- Dolichoectasia may cause ischemic strokes, hemorrhagic strokes, cranial nerve deficits, brainstem compression, and hydrocephalus.
- Potential mechanisms for ischemic stroke include hemodynamic, intraluminal thrombus occluding the opening of brainstem branch arteries, artery-to-artery embolism, small vessel ischemic disease, and dissection.
- The optimal non-invasive imaging techniques are CTA and MRA with contrast. Conventional angiography remains the gold standard.
- Prognosis is highly variable ranging from asymptomatic or few deficits to severe deficits. Recurrent ischemia is much more common than recurrent intracranial hemorrhage.
- The best treatment approach remains unclear. Antiplatelets or ant-icoagulation are often used. However, caution is recommended in giving antiplatelets or anticoagulation to patients who present with non-ischemic symptoms (i.e., cranial nerve deficits).

Further Reading

Anson JA, Lawton MT, Spetzler RF. (1996). Characteristics and surgical treatment of dolichoectatic and fusiform aneuryms. *J Neurosurg* 84:185-193.

Passero SG, Calchetti B, Bartalini S. (2005). Intracranial bleeding in patients with vertebrobasilar dolichoectasia. *Stroke* 36: 1421-1425.

Passero SG, Rossi S. (2008). Natural history of vertebrobasilar dolichoectasia. *Neurology* 70:66-72.

Pico F, Labreuche J, Touboul P-J, Leys D, Amarenco P. (2003). Intracranial arterial dolichoectasia and its relation with atherosclerosis and stroke subtype. *Neurology* 61:1736-1742.

Pico F, Labreuche J, Touboul P-J, Leys D, Amarenco P. (2005). Intracranial arterial dolichoectasia and small-vessel disease in stroke patients. *Ann Neurol* 57:472-479.

Savitz S, Caplan LR. (2008). Dilatative arteriopathy (dolichoectasia) in Uncommon Causes of stroke 2nd ed, Caplan LR (Ed) New York, Cambridge University Press pp 479-482.

Savitz S, Ronthal M, Caplan LR. (2006). Vertebral artery compression of the medulla. *Arch Neurol* 63:234-241.

22 Arteriovenous Malformations

A 40-year-old woman had 2 generalized convulsions while at work. Emergency medical technicians (EMTs) found her postictal and normotensive; she was brought to a hospital emergency department. There, noncontrast head CT showed a right parieto-occipital intraparenchymal hemorrhage without surrounding edema. She was loaded with phenytoin and admitted to the neurology service.

On questioning, the woman admits to having occasional, severe right posterior headaches over the past several months. She denies health problems or drug abuse and she takes no medications. Neurological examination was normal except for a left homonymous hemianopia and visual neglect of the left side of pictures and objects.

The next morning, the patient had an MRI and MRA that showed a 4cm right parieto-occipital arteriovenous malformation (AVM) with an associated large draining vein; there was also evidence of past bleeding.

What do you do now?

Arteriovenous malformations are the most dangerous cerebral vascular malformation. They are congenital, sporadic developmental vascular lesions, with an estimated overall incidence of 0.1%; the incidence is higher in people with hereditary hemorrhagic telangiectasia (i.e., Osler-Weber-Rendu syndrome). The majority of these lesions are supratentorial.

AVMs are characterized by direct arterial to venous connection without a normal intervening capillary network; gliotic brain may be admixed with the vascular tangle, and calcifications are often present. The high-flow communication may cause formation of pedicle aneurysms and arterialization of the venous limb. The most feared complication is hemorrhage. Local parenchymal perfusion may occasionally be compromised due to a "flow stealing" phenomenon; correspondingly, there is microscopic evidence of chronic ischemia and gliosis in the brain tissue adjacent to the AVM.

AVMs generally become symptomatic between the ages of 10 years and 40 years; presentations range from headache to seizure to hemorrhage. Some have summarized the symptoms as "they ache (headache), break (bleed), and shake (have seizures)." Intracranial hemorrhage on presentation is the strongest predictor for subsequent hemorrhage if the AVM is left untreated. Other risk factors for hemorrhage include advanced age, deep venous drainage pattern, deep brain location, and associated aneurysms.

Diagnostic evaluation usually starts with noncontrast head CT. This will either show hemorrhage (if it has occurred) or a cluster of calcifications and hyperattenuated vascular channels. MRI clarifies the extent of the AVM, identifies the associated draining veins, and may show signs of past bleeding related to the lesion. Conventional angiography is the gold standard for diagnosis and treatment planning. It gives invaluable information on nidus configuration, relationship to neighboring vessels, and localization of the draining portion; any associated aneurysms are also clearly defined.

Controversy surrounds the question of which patients with AVMs should be treated. Most clinicians and researchers agree that once an AVM bleeds it should be treated to prevent further bleeding if treatment is feasible. Treatment may involve direct surgical removal at craniotomy, interventional obliteration through the arterial or venous systems, and/or methods of focal targeted irradiation or combinations of these modalities. Treatment often involves cooperation and collaboration among multiple specialists.

A case series and a nonrandomized population-based report suggest that treatment of nonruptured AVMs is associated with worse outcome than no treatment. A randomized controlled trial comparing medical management of unruptured brain AVMs and invasive treatment (i.e., any combination of surgery, radiosurgery, and endovascular embolization) is ongoing.

In an attempt to identify those patients who would benefit most from surgical intervention, a formula has been devised. This calculation takes into account patient age and annual risk of hemorrhage to give an estimate of cumulative hemorrhage risk:

$$\text{Lifetime risk of hemorrhage} = 1 - (1-P)^N$$

N = expected years of life remaining
P = annual probability of hemorrhage.

Surgical risk assessment has most often been based on the Spetzler-Martin Grading Scale (Table 22.1). This scale assigns points based on the size, location, and venous drainage pattern of the AVM in question.

Our patient had conventional dye-contrast angiography—and, based on those results—is given a Spetzler-Martin Grade of II. Given that her expected years of life remaining is 40 and her annual probability of hemorrhage is estimated at 3%, she has an extremely high lifetime risk of hemorrhage. Surgery is recommended in her case.

TABLE 22.1 **Spetzler-Martin Grading Scale for AVMs**

CHARACTERISTIC	NUMBER OF POINTS
Size of AVM	
Small (<3cm)	1 point
Medium (3-6cm)	2 points
Large (>6cm)	3 points
Location	
Non-eloquent site	0 points
Eloquent site	1 point
Pattern of Venous Drainage	
Superficial only	0 points
Deep component	1 point

- AVMs are the most dangerous cerebral vascular malformation and have an incidence of 0.1%.
- AVMs are characterized by direct arterial-venous connections and may include aneurysms; adjacent brain is often gliotic.
- Risk factors for subsequent hemorrhage include hemorrhage on presentation, advanced age, deep venous drainage pattern, deep brain location, and associated aneurysms.
- Conventional angiography is the gold standard for diagnosis and treatment planning.
- Intervention remains controversial, but is generally recommended for surgically accessible lesions in patients with high lifetime risk of hemorrhage.

Further Reading

Al-Shahi R, Warlow C. (2001). A systematic review of the frequency and prognosis of arteriovenous malformations of the brain in adults. *Brain* 124:1900-1926.

Brown RD Jr. (2008). Unruptured brain AVMs: to treat or not to treat. *Lancet Neurol* 7:195-196.

Choi JH, Mast H, Sciacca RR, et al. (2006). Clinical outcome after first and recurrent hemorrhage in patients with untreated brain arteriovenous malformation. *Stroke* 37:1243-1247.

Cockroft KM. (2007). Unruptured brain arteriovenous malformations should be treated conservatively: no. *Stroke* 38:3310-3311.

da Costa L, Wallace MC, Ter Brugge KG, et al. (2009). The natural history and predictive features of hemorrhage from brain arteriovenous malformations. *Stroke* 40:100-105.

Davis SM, Donnan GA. (2007). Unruptured brain arteriovenous malformations: another asymptomatic conundrum. *Stroke* 38:3312.

Friedlander RM. (2007). Clinical practice: arteriovenous malformations of the brain. *N Engl J Med* 356:2704-2712.

Kaibara T, Heros RC. (2008). Arteriovenous malformations of the brain. In: *Uncommon Causes of Stroke*, 2nd edition (Caplan LR, ed.), pp 181-188. Cambridge UK, Cambridge University Press.

Khaw AV, Mohr JP, Sciacca RR, et al. (2004). Association of infratentorial brain arteriovenous malformations with hemorrhage at initial presentation. *Stroke* 35:660.

McCormick WF. (1984). Pathology of vascular malformations of the brain. In: *Intracranial Arteriovenous Malformations* (Wilson CB, Stein BM, eds.), p. 44. Baltimore, MD, William & Wilkins.

Spetzler RF, Martin NA. (1986). A proposed grading system for arteriovenous malformations. *J Neurosurg* 65:476–483.

Stapf C, Mast H, Sciacca RR, et al. (2006). Predictors of hemorrhage in patients with untreated brain arteriovenous malformation. *Neurology* 66:1350–1355.

Stapf C, Mohr JP. (2007). Unruptured brain arteriovenous malformations should be treated conservatively. *Stroke* 38:3308–3309.

Wedderburn CJ, van Beijnum J, Bhattacharya JJ, et al. (2008). Outcome after interventional or conservative management of unruptured brain arteriovenous malformations: a prospective, population-based cohort study. *Lancet Neurol* 7:223–230.

23 Cavernous Angiomas

A 35-year-old right-handed man was referred for evaluation and management of a recent transient ischemic attack (TIA). He woke up one morning complaining of clumsiness of the right hand and arm. He had no other neurological symptoms. He was evaluated in an outside hospital. His clumsiness improved spontaneously a few hours later. His work-up included: 1) a head CT scan, which was negative; 2) carotid Doppler, which was unrevealing; 3) TTE/TEE transthoracic echocardiography/transesophageal echocardiography, which showed the presence of a patent foramen ovale with right-to-left shunt; and 4) lower extremity Doppler ultrasound and hypercoagulability panel, which were all negative. His cardiologist advised him to take warfarin for a presumptive TIA due to paradoxical embolism. His neurologist, however, recommended aspirin. Therefore, he sought a second opinion. He was overall healthy. He never smoked or used recreational drugs. His medications only included warfarin. On examination, blood pressure was 110/70; pulse was 76 beats per minute and regular. His neurological examination was entirely normal.

What do you do now?

Although TIA was clearly a concern, the lack of speech or language involvement was somewhat atypical for a cardioembolic event and raised the possibility of focal seizure as a differential diagnosis. Brain MRI with and without gadolinium and MRA were ordered to complete his evaluation. His MRI revealed a lesion in the mid-left frontal lobe (Fig 23.1). The overall appearance of the lesion was consistent with a cavernous malformation (CM). Warfarin was discontinued, and the patient opted not to take prophylactic antiseizure medications. A year later, he reported brief episodes of word finding difficulties on a daily basis. He was started on levetiracetam for presumptive focal seizures. A repeat MRI suggested new bleeding in his CM during this interval.

Cerebral cavernous malformation, also known as cavernous angioma or cavernoma, is characterized by an abnormal cluster of blood vessels embedded in normal brain tissue and enclosed in a capsule. Cavernous malformations account for approximately 5% to 13% of all vascular malformations. They lack the high flow arterial feeders and draining veins of typical arteriovenous malformations. Pathologically, CM is comprised of multiple sinusoid-like capillary channels containing blood in a sluggish circulation and lined by a single-layered endothelium, which is prone to leaking. There is no neural tissue in these walls but the periphery is surrounded by a pseudocapsule of gliotic brain. Cavernous malformations are often small, but may enlarge due to recurrent bleeding and clot organization.

Most cases of CM are sporadic; familial cavernomas occur in 20% to 50% of all cases. Three genes have been linked to familial cavernous malformations; CCM1 on chromosome 7 in Hispanics, CCM2 on chromosome 7, and CCM3 on chromosome 3. Multiple CM may occur in up to 30% of sporadic cases, and in up to 80% of familial cases. CMs may involve any brain or spinal region and are most often found within the cerebral hemispheres, pons, and cerebellum. CMs are often accompanied by developmental venous anomalies (DVAs), and some CMs develop years after cranial irradiation.

Brain CMs are often occult, i.e., not evident on neurological examination. Approximately 25% of individuals with CM will never develop any related symptoms. When symptoms develop, they usually occur between the second and fourth decades. The usual presenting symptoms are: seizure,

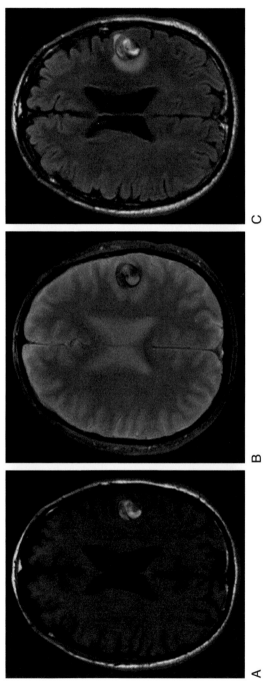

FIGURE 23.1 Brain MRI reveals a round heterogeneous hyperintense lesion on T1 (image A) with areas of T2* susceptibility (image B) consistent with hemorrhage and mild surrounding edema on FLAIR (image C). The lesion has a "popcorn" or "honeycomb" appearance, which is characteristic of a cavernous malformation.

headache, progressive neurological deficit, or brain hemorrhage. Seizures are the most common symptom and are reported in up to 70% of patients. They are most often focal in nature, although many will secondarily generalize. The exact mechanisms by which CMs cause seizures are not clear. It is speculated that the breakdown products caused by repeated microhemorrhages deposit ferric iron into the surrounding cortex, which is epileptogenic.

Cerebral CMs are often detected during evaluation of patients with a first seizure. CMs identified on imaging studies may be incidental without a role in seizure onset in approximately 6% of cases. The diagnosis is mostly straightforward with the use of modern MRI imaging techniques. MRI is usually diagnostic and shows a well-circumscribed intraparenchymal lesion with a heterogeneous core of mixed signal intensity and a surrounding rim of low signal intensity. The mixed signal intensity within the center represents small hemorrhages of different ages, and the surrounding rim represents hemosiderin in the surrounding cortex. Although the imaging appearance of CM on MRI is quite characteristic, large cavernomas may form a cystic growth mimicking a neoplasm. Angiography is rarely necessary because the lesions do not have high flow arterial feeders or anomalous drainage, and are usually not shown. On CT scan, CM may appear as nonspecific hyperdensities, often thought to be "calcifications."

Brain parenchymatous hemorrhage is the most feared complication of cerebral CM. The reported incidence of hemorrhage varies from 8% to 37% in adults in different series. However, the risk of hemorrhage overall is believed to be relatively small, varying from 0.4% to 0.6% per year; and is higher in patients that have previously bled. The risk of hemorrhage is cumulative over the life expectancy of the patient, and is therefore of more concern in younger patients. Despite the significant deficits that can develop after hemorrhage from a CM, patients often improve dramatically over time. Hemorrhages are most often contained within the capsule of the CM and rarely drain into surrounding brain parenchyma, or the ventricles or subarachnoid space. Repeated hemorrhages, however, can cause enlargement of a CM and a stepwise neurological deterioration.

The therapeutic strategy for brain CMs must be guided by the size of the lesion, its location, whether it is symptomatic or not, and the risk it imparts to the patient. Incidental and asymptomatic lesions should be observed.

The decision is relatively easy in patients who present with a first seizure, and mostly relies on the use of antiepileptic medications for seizure control. In patients with CMs and chronic intractable seizures, management should be guided by the benefit/risk ratio of further anticonvulsant therapy vs. the benefit/risk ratio of surgical excision. The current indications for treatment of CM are recurrent bleeding, progressive neurological deficit, or intractable epilepsy. Treatment options include: surgical resection or stereotactic radiosurgery. The location of the lesion in the vicinity of an eloquent cortical region such as the language areas of the brain and its association with another venous anomaly are associated with increased surgical risks including residual neurological injury and venous infarction. It is also important to consider that: 1) resection of the CM does not necessarily relieve the patients of their seizures for a variety of reasons, including postoperative scar formation; 2) the prospective natural history of cerebral CM and optimal management strategy are ill-defined, and are currently under prospective investigations.

In our patient, the lesion was not amenable to endovascular intervention. Given the location of his lesion, he underwent functional MRI of the brain to delineate the speech area in order to further assess his surgical risk, which showed activation posterior to the lesion. He successfully underwent surgical excision of the lesion without persistent complications.

KEY POINTS TO REMEMBER

- Brain and vascular imaging are important in patients with brain ischemia even when the clinical symptoms/signs are transient.
- Patent foramen ovale and cavernous angiomas are often incidental findings unrelated to the clinical syndrome.
- Cavernomas are abnormal clusters of sinusoidal capillaries embedded in normal brain tissue.
- The most frequent associated symptom in patients with cavernomas is seizures.
- Hemorrhage can be recurrent, but blood is usually contained within the capsule of the lesion.

- Treatment depends heavily on the nature and seriousness of the symptoms, the location and size of the lesions, and the benefit/ risk ratio of medical treatment vs. surgical or radiosurgical obliteration.

Further Reading

Ebrahimi A, Etemadifar M, Ardestani PM, Maghzi AH, Jaffe S, Nejadnik H. (2009). Cavernous angioma: a clinical study of 35 cases with review of the literature. *Neurol Res*. 31:785-793.

Kondziolka D, Lunsford LD, Kestle JR. (1995). The natural history of cerebral cavernous malformations. *J Neurosurg* 83:820-824.

Leblanc GG, Golanov E, Awad IA, Young WL. (2009). Biology of Vascular Malformations of the Brain NINDS Workshop Collaborators. Biology of vascular malformations of the brain. *Stroke* 40:e694-702.

McLaughlin MR, Kondziolka D, Flickinger JC, Lunsford S, Lunsford LD. (1998). The prospective natural history of cerebral venous malformations. *Neurosurgery* 43:195-200.

Metellus C, Kharkar S, Lin D, Kapoor S, Rigamonti D. (2008). Cerebral cavernous malformations and developmental venous anomalies in Uncommon causes of stroke 2nd ed, Caplan LR, (Ed) pp 189-220.

Rigamonti D. (2008). In: *Uncommon Causes of Stroke*, 2nd edition (Caplan LR, ed.), Cambridge, UK, Cambridge University Press.

24 Post-Cardiac Surgery Encephalopathy and Stroke

You are called to provide consultation for a 74-year-old man who remains agitated and confused after coronary artery bypass performed 5 days before. He has had hypertension for 30 years that has been relatively well controlled. He also is overweight and has had diabetes for 10 years. He has had lower extremity vascular bypass surgery to treat claudication. Because of increasing angina he had coronary angiography that showed severe 3-vessel coronary artery disease. Aspirin was discontinued a week before surgery. A coronary artery bypass graft (CABG) procedure was performed without obvious complications. After surgery he was slow to awaken and when he did stir he became hyperactive and has been given increasing doses of haloperidol. Atorvastatin (given in 80 mg/evening dose preoperatively) had not been restarted after surgery.

Examination shows a restrained man. Pulse 82 and regular, blood pressure 145/85. No neck bruits. He mumbles incoherent replies to queries and does not follow commands reliably. He moves his right arm and both legs more than his left arm and deep tendon reflexes are exaggerated on the left. Both plantar responses are extensor.

An MRI scan shows a scattering of small infarcts, mostly in the border-zone regions of the cerebral and cerebellar hemispheres. A slightly larger infarct involves the parasylvian right cerebral convexity surface.

What do you do now?

This patient has developed strokes and encephalopathy related to cardiac surgery. Haloperidol use likely adds to his encephalopathy and should be stopped. Haloperidol is very slowly removed from the circulation. Its use substantially delays recovery. When patients develop rebound hyperactivity on withdrawing from haloperidol, physicians unfortunately often prescribe an even higher dose. In my opinion haloperidol should never be used in older patients, especially in those with neurological abnormalities. The one indication is hemiballism when other measures do not control the violent motions. Cessation of statins can lead to a rebound increase in the likelihood of cardiac and brain ischemic events. I prescribed beginning again atorvastatin 80 mg/day given through his nasogastric tube.

The major causes of stroke and encephalopathy after coronary artery bypass graft (CABG) relate to emboli emanating from the heart and the aorta. Decreased ventricular and atrial contractility and postoperative atrial fibrillation are important causes of stroke. The most important risk factor for stroke after cardiopulmonary bypass surgery is aortic atheromas. Some patients have very atherosclerotic aortas with protruding atheromas (Fig 24.1). Low mean arterial blood pressure and prolonged bypass time increase the likelihood of the patient developing strokes and encephalopathy postoperatively.

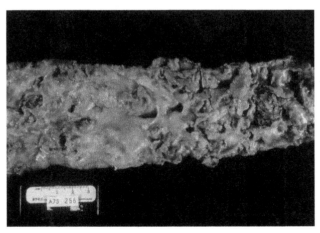

FIGURE 24.1   A very atherosclerotic aorta at necropsy. From *Brain Embolism* (Caplan LR, Manning WJ, eds.), New York, Informa Healthcare, 2006, with permission.

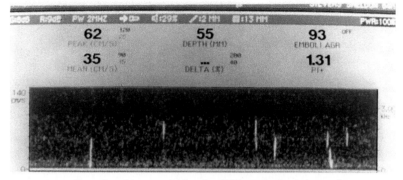

FIGURE 24.2 Recording of transcranial Doppler (TCD) monitoring during cardiac surgery when the aorta was first clamped. The white linear regions represent high-intensity transient signals indicative of microemboli passing the MCA. From *Brain Embolism* (Caplan LR, Manning WJ, eds.), New York, Informa Healthcare, 2006, with permission.

Preoperative transesophageal echocardiography can detect atrial and ventricular dysfunction and can localize and quantify the presence of aortic plaques and protruding atheromas. Unfortunately this patient did not have echocardiography before surgery.

Transcranial Doppler (TCD) monitoring during maneuvers that involve manipulation of atheromatous aortas, such as cannulation and clamping and unclamping, often show large numbers of microemboli emanating from the aorta. Figure 24.2 is a TCD recording taken during aortic clamping showing many small white high-intensity transient signals (HITS) that indicate microemboli. At times the numbers of microemboli are so numerous that a "white out" of emboli occurs.

When severe aortic atherosclerosis is detected preoperatively or even at surgery using a hand-held Doppler, a number of alternatives arise: using "off-pump" surgery, pump-assisted bypass without cross-clamping the aorta, clamping at a location relatively free of disease, or instituting a filter placed in the aorta to catch embolic debris. None of these strategies were used in this patient.

Cessation of haloperidol resulted in the patient awakening rather completely and rapidly. Only reassurance and nursing supervision were needed to calm the agitation. Examination after awakening revealed a very slight left hemiparesis and poor memory and visual-spatial functions. These abnormalities improved but prevented him from returning to his job as a surveyor. A transesophageal echocardiogram showed regions of decreased ventricular mobility, an ejection fraction of 35%, and a very atherosclerotic aorta with protruding plaques. Antiplatelet therapy was also reinstituted, but there seemed not to be an indication for prophylactic anticoagulation.

Economic concerns have led payors to dictate that patients having elective coronary artery bypass surgery be admitted to the hospital on the day of surgery. Although most have had coronary artery angiography, many have not had an adequate assessment of atrial and ventricular function, or echocardiographic study of their hearts and their aortas for the presence of thrombi and aortic atheromas. Physicians must push for adequate preoperative studies. These will likely save lives and brain tissue.

KEY POINTS TO REMEMBER

- Haloperidol should not be used in older patients, especially those with abnormal brains.
- The most common cause of strokes and encephalopathy after coronary artery bypass surgery is embolization from atherosclerotic aortic atheromas.
- Thorough evaluation including a history of transient ischemic attacks and strokes, and studies of cardiac function and aortic atherosclerosis should precede elective coronary artery bypass surgery
- Strategies for surgery—on-pump vs. off-pump, and management of the aorta should be planned before surgery

Further Reading

Barbut D, Yao FS, Hager DN, et al. (1996). Comparison of transcranial Doppler ultrasonography and transesophageal echocardiography during coronary artery bypass surgery. *Stroke* 27:87-90.

Barbut D, Caplan LR. (1997). Brain complications of cardiac surgery. *Curr Probl Cardiol* 22:447-476.

Caplan LR. (2009). (Editorial) Translating what is known about neurological complications of coronary artery bypass graft surgery into action. *Arch Neurol* 66(9):1062-1064.

Caplan LR. (2006). The aorta as a donor source of brain embolism. In *Brain Embolism* (Caplan LR, Manning WJ, eds.), pp. 187-201. New York, Informa Healthcare.

Mackensen GB, Ti LK, Phillips-Bute BG, et al.; Neurologic Outcome Research Group (NORG). (2003). Cerebral embolization during cardiac surgery: impact of aortic atheroma burden. *Br J Anesth* 91:656-661.

Bacterial Endocarditis

A 62-year-old man is brought to the emergency room after being found roaming the hallways of his apartment building. He lives alone and was last seen well by neighbors two days before. He was unable to provide a cogent history but was recognized by staff from prior evaluations. Previous medical history was notable for hypertension, cirrhosis due to chronic alcohol use, alcohol intoxication with withdrawal seizures, tobacco use, and medication noncompliance.

On examination, he was febrile with oral temperature 101.4°F. Blood pressure was elevated at 150/95 and heart was regular at 92 bpm. He had superficial abrasions and ecchymoses on his left forehead, volar surfaces of his hands, and right elbow. There was a holosystolic murmur. Lungs were clear. Abdomen was slightly tender in the left upper quadrant but without rebound tenderness. He was alert but inattentive. He would give his name and follow single-step commands but language was impaired. Spontaneous speech was sparse, as the patient indicated that he was "feeling sick." He could not name or repeat. Fundoscopic exam was normal. Pupils were symmetric and reactive. His eyes moved conjugately but were deviated to the right at rest. Visual fields were full. Smile was symmetric. Appendicular strength was intact. Reflexes were symmetric, plantar responses were flexor. There was a subtle pronator drift of the right arm. Sensation was intact and he did not extinguish to double simultaneous stimulation. He had no dysmetria or dysdiadochokinesia. The patient walked without assistance, albeit with discomfort.

He had a noncontrast head CT that showed subtle hypodensities in the left temporal and right frontal regions consistent with subacute brain infarcts. Chest radiograph was normal. His white blood count (WBC) was elevated at 18,900/mcL. PT/INR and aPTT were normal. Serum chemistries were suggestive of acute kidney injury with a serum creatinine of 1.9mg/dL. EKG showed sinus tachycardia. Blood cultures were drawn, and the patient was admitted.

Brain MRI showed acute infarcts in the left temporal and right frontal lobes and a few scattered foci in the right cerebellum. No associated hemorrhage was found. A proximal, embolic source was suspected. The patient remained febrile in spite of antipyretic medications. Abdominal CT was performed for renal failure and abdominal pain and showed splenic and renal infarcts. Blood cultures grew out gram positive cocci identified as Methicillin-resistant Staphylococcus aureus (MRSA). Because of persistent fever, new murmur, and MRSA bacteremia, endocarditis was strongly suspected.

Transthoracic echocardiogram was normal.
A transesophageal echocardiogram was performed and revealed a 1.2 x 0.9 cm mobile vegetation on the posterior leaflet of the mitral valve.

Antiplatelets or anticoagulants were not administered. After initiation of vancomycin, the patient defervesced and began to improve clinically. A follow up brain MRI one week later showed no additional infarcts.

What do you do now?

Endocarditis remains a clinically challenging and potentially devastating diagnosis. As epidemiology and culprit organisms evolve, atypical presentations, often subtle in early stages, make diagnosis a challenge. As stroke or other systemic embolization are the feared complications, the importance of an early diagnosis cannot be overstated. The Duke criteria, among others used, incorporate historical factors, clinical examination findings, and diagnostic tests, chiefly echocardiography. Risk factors can be grouped as risks of infection (HIV infection, immunosuppressive state or medication use), risks of bacteremia (intravenous drug use, indwelling catheters, chronic hemodialysis), and risks of cardiac valvular abnormalities (prosthetic heart valves, Rheumatic fever, prior history of endocarditis). Classic clinical findings include fever and mucocutaneous embolization (Roth spots, Janeway lesions, Osler's nodes). The *sine qua non* of endocarditis is the presence of cardiac valvular vegetations on echocardiography. Often, the transesophageal approach, particularly for adequate view of posterior leaflets and small vegetations, proves more sensitive than transthoracic approach. Epidemiologically the mitral valve, followed by aortic, tricuspid and pulmonic valves are most often affected.

The microbiology of endocarditis has implications not only in choosing appropriate antimicrobial therapy but also in predicting the likelihood of systemic complications as well as to identify organisms associated with atypical presentations. Staphylococci and streptococci represent the most common species implicated. Embolization is more common in Staphylococcus infections. A subset of patients with endocarditis will harbor difficult-to-culture organisms, usually gram negative bacilli *Haemophilus* species., *Actinobacillus actinomycetemcomitans*, *Cardiobacterium hominis*, *Eikenella corrodens* and *Kingella* species-organisms (HACEK), Coxiella and Bartonella among the more common), which could delay diagnosis and increase the risk of complications.

Endocarditis is a relatively uncommon cause of stroke, but stroke in patients with endocarditis is fairly common, clinically apparent in over 1/3 of patients but asymptomatically present in another 50%. Several factors are implicated in the likelihood of embolization. Larger vegetations, ones on the mitral and to less extent aortic valve, and ones from *Staphylococcus aureus* carry higher risks. Smaller or streptococcal vegetations still can cause emboli, as can vegetations in the right heart. Lastly, the presence of positive phospholipid antibodies are thrombophilic markers increasing the risk of embolization.

Traditionally, treatment of "cardioembolic stroke" is anticoagulation. However, in embolic stroke from endocarditis, anticoagulation is not routinely given, because of the increased risk of hemorrhage. If the patient had been on anticoagulants (e.g., because of a prosthetic valve or atrial fibrillation with a large left atrium), then they are continued. Likewise, anti-platelet agents are unlikely to confer additional benefit but will increase hemorrhagic risk (albeit less than anticoagulation). Risk with anticoagulation is further increased by the possibility of the rare complication of a mycotic aneurysm—arterial wall erosion and dilatations from invasion of infective agent. The mainstay of treatment is appropriate antimicrobial therapy. Additionally, in patients with embolization (whether cranial or systemic), screening for occult embolization after initiation of antimicrobial therapy can be useful. Recurrent infarction several days after the initiation of appropriate antimicrobial therapy is an indication for valvular surgery as it suggests medical failure. Cerebral hemorrhage or vascular imaging that suggest aneurysm formation requires a formal angiogram for diagnosis and possible treatment of a mycotic aneurysm.

KEY POINTS TO REMEMBER

- Transesophageal approach to echocardiography is more sensitive than transthoracic approach.
- Vegetations can be the source for systemic (e.g., splenic or renal) as well as cerebral emboli and infarction.
- Anticoagulation is usually not indicated in endocarditis complicated by stroke.
- Treatment is with antimicrobials.
- Recurrent embolization after initiation of appropriate antimicrobial therapy is an indication for consideration of valvular surgery.

Further Reading

Caplan LR, Manning WJ. Cardiac sources of embolism. In: *Brain Embolism* (Caplan LR, Manning WJ, eds.), pp. 129–186. New York, Informa Healthcare.

Chan KL, Dumesnil JG, Cujec B, Sanfilippo AJ, Jue J, Turek MA, Robinson TI, Moher D; Investigators of the Multicenter Aspirin Study in Infective Endocarditis. (2003). A randomized trial of aspirin on the risk of embolic events in patients with infective endocarditis. *J Am Coll Cardiol* 42:775-780.

Dickerman SA, Abrutyn E, Barsic B, et. al. (2007). The relationship between the initiation of antimicrobial therapy and the incidence of stroke in infective endocarditis: an analysis from the ICE prospective cohort study. *Am Heart J* 154:1086-1094.

Durack DT, Lukes AS, Bright DK. (1994). New criteria for diagnosis of infective endocarditis: utilization of specific echocardiographic findings. *Am J Med* 96: 200-209.

Jones HR, Siekert RG. (1989). Neurological manifestations of infective endocarditis. Review of clinical and therapeutic challenges. *Brain* 112:1295-1315.

Tornos P, Almirante B, Mirabet S, Permanyer G, Pahissa A, Soler-Soler J. (1999). Infective endocarditis due to *Staphylococcus aureus*: deleterious effect of anticoagulant therapy. *Arch Intern Med* 159:473-475.

26 Coexistent Severe Coronary and Carotid Artery Disease

A 68-year-old woman with hypertension and diabetes is admitted with substernal chest pain and dyspnea on exertion for the last week. She had coronary angiography that revealed severe 3-vessel coronary artery disease. The cardiovascular surgeon evaluated the patient and recommended coronary artery bypass graft (CABG) surgery. Before the procedure the surgeon noted a left carotid bruit and ordered an ultrasound examination of the neck arteries. The Doppler examination was consistent with 60% stenosis of the left internal carotid artery and less than 30% stenosis of the right. The patient denied any prior history or symptoms suggestive of TIA or stroke. The cardiovascular surgeon wishes to know what effect the carotid stenosis will have on the patient's operative risk. In addition, the surgeon asks if performing carotid endarterectomy prior to CABG will help to minimize the patient's stroke risk.

What do you do now?

Stroke after coronary artery bypass graft (CABG) is a major cause of operative mortality and morbidity. Patients who have stroke after surgery have longer hospitalizations and a higher risk of long-term disability. Perioperative stroke occurs in about 1.4–3.8% of CABG surgeries. Approximately 30–40% of these are detected in the immediate postoperative period, while the rest are found after the patient awakens from anesthesia uneventfully. The mechanism of the majority of perioperative strokes is embolism from the heart or aorta. Although hypoperfusion is often a concern intra-operatively, it accounted for only 9% of strokes in a series of 388 patients in northern New England who had CABG surgery.

Risk factors for perioperative stroke include advanced age, history of hypertension, congestive heart failure, diabetes, and peripheral vascular disease. Aortic atherosclerosis is a major risk for perioperative stroke and encephalopathy. The risk of stroke during CABG is high in those patients who have had past strokes and have symptomatic carotid artery disease but is low in patients with asymptomatic carotid artery disease. It is important to identify patients with symptomatic disease and those in whom carotid artery disease has caused strokes shown by brain imaging. This is accomplished through careful inquiry about symptoms suggestive of stroke or transient ischemic attacks (TIAs), the presence of which should prompt further neurovascular and brain imaging.

Patients with asymptomatic carotid artery stenosis are often identified preoperatively by auscultation of a carotid bruit. Carotid bruits are present in about 10% of patients undergoing CABG surgery. The presence of a carotid bruit does not correlate with the degree of underlying stenosis nor does it correlate with the risk of perioperative stroke. Carotid bruits are associated with long-term risk of stroke during the following years. Often the stroke is in a territory incongruent with the affected vessel, suggesting that the presence of a bruit is a marker for atherosclerosis and stroke risk in general.

In contrast to patients with symptomatic carotid artery stenosis, the reported risk of stroke in patients with asymptomatic carotid disease has varied widely, with some studies showing an increased risk while others have not. This discrepancy is largely due to the varying nature of the studies that have addressed this issue, and so uncertainty as to the significance of asymptomatic carotid stenosis remains. The bulk of the available evidence however, suggests that patients with stenosis less than 70% are not at significantly increased risk of perioperative stroke after CABG. Contralateral carotid artery occlusion may be a risk factor for perioperative stroke but is not amenable to revascularization.

The question posed by this case scenario concerns the benefits of prophylactically revascularizing patients with asymptomatic carotid stenosis before or during CABG surgery. Patients with recently symptomatic coronary artery disease were excluded from carotid surgery trials and therefore prospective data on the risks and benefits of carotid endarterectomy (CE) in these patients is lacking. There is no convincing evidence that combining CE and CABG reduces postoperative stroke risk. Most perioperative strokes are not preventable by revascularization as they are attributable to causes other than carotid stenosis. In a recent study, among over 3900 patients who had CABG surgery, 95% (72 of 76 patients) had strokes not related to carotid artery disease. Time is better directed toward evaluating patients for aortic atherosclerotic and poor cardiac function, as these are more common sources of embolism. Adjusting surgical technique accordingly in these patients may improve outcome. Some data suggest harm to the patient undergoing revascularization at the same time as CABG as combined carotid and coronary surgery has a higher risk than that attributable to the sum of the two procedures and morbidity of the combined procedures is higher than each individual surgery. Some cardiac surgeons favor carotid artery surgery or stenting before or during CABG in patients with asymptomatic carotid disease who have stenosis >80% or bilateral severe stenosis, but there is no evidence-base for this approach.

The risk may be unaffected by the timing of the surgery. Two general approaches to revascularization are concomitant CE and CABG versus a staged CE prior to or after CABG approach. Recently an expert panel of the American Academy of Neurology reviewed the available data concerning timing of CE and CABG. They reported an overall perioperative stroke rate of 3% for patients who have combined CE-CABG based on 9 studies totaling 1923 patients. Death and myocardial infarction (MI) rates were 4.7% and 2.2% respectively. For staged CE prior to CABG the stroke rate based on 1 study evaluating 257 patients was 1.9%, while death and MI rates were 1.6% and 4.7%. Based on these findings, the panel concluded that there is no evidence to declare a superior approach.

Carotid artery stenting (CAS) is increasingly becoming available as a less invasive alternative to CE. However, the benefits of CAS prior to CABG remain uncertain. A recent systematic review of 6 studies including 277 patients undergoing CAS prior to CABG found a 30-day risk of any stroke or death of 12.3% for the combined procedures. In this report only a fraction of the patients undergoing CAS were treated with distal protection devices to prevent embolization. Further studies using higher rates of distal protection will be needed to further clarify the role of stenting in patients undergoing CABG. In addition, hemodynamic studies employing transcranial Doppler ultrasound, CT, or MR perfusion studies may prove valuable in identifying patients with hemodynamically significant carotid artery stenosis who are at increased risk of perioperative stroke; however at present the benefit of their routine clinical use has not been studied.

KEY POINTS TO REMEMBER

- Most patients with asymptomatic carotid stenosis undergoing CABG are not at an increased risk of perioperative stroke.
- The most common mechanism of perioperative stroke in patients with carotid stenosis is embolism from the heart or aorta. Only a small percentage of strokes are caused by hypoperfusion.
- Perioperative stroke is most often recognized after a delay from anesthesia recovery.
- Routine revascularization of patients with carotid stenosis is not warranted in patients undergoing CABG as it exposes the patient to the risks associated with two procedures.
- Detailed preoperative evaluation that includes a thorough history and examination, and assessment of cardiac function and the presence and extent of aortic atheromas can help with planning of CABG surgery and should reduce stroke incidence, morbidity, and mortality after CABG surgery.

Further Reading

Bucerius J, Gummert JF, Borger MA, et al. (2003). Stroke after cardiac surgery: a risk factor analysis of 16,184 consecutive adult patients. *Ann Thorac Surg* 75:472-478.

Caplan LR. (2009). (Editorial) Translating what is known about neurological complications of coronary artery bypass graft surgery into action. *Arch Neurol* 66(9):1062-1064.

Das SK, Brow TD, Pepper J. (2000). Continuing controversy in the management of concomitant coronary and carotid disease: an overview. *Int J Cardiol* 74:47-65.

Guzman LA, Costa MA, Angiolillo DJ, et al. (2008). A systematic review of outcomes in patients with staged carotid artery stenting and coronary artery bypass graft surgery. *Stroke* 39:361-365.

Li Y, Walicki D, Mathiesen C, et al. (2009). Strokes following open heart surgery aren't related to carotid stenosis. *Arch Neurol* 66:1091-1096.

Likosky DS, Marrin CA, Caplan LR, et al. (2003). Determination of etiologic mechanisms of strokes secondary to coronary artery bypass graft surgery. *Stroke* 34:2830-2834.

Index

Note: Page references followed by '*f*' and '*t*' denote figures and tables respectively.